DICTIONARY OF MEDICAL EMERGENCIES
English - Croatian

RJEČNIK HITNIH MEDICINSKIH INTERVENCIJA
Englesko – Hrvatski

Edita Ciglenečki

INTRODUCTION - UVOD

The audience for this dictionary includes medical professionals working in multilingual environments; global health professionals in tourist areas; professionals in public health, humanitarian medicine, emergency disaster management, rescue teams and above all, frequent travellers disposed to any kind of danger or health risk and therefore in the need of medical assistance while in some foreign speaking country. In emergency situations even small misunderstandings can lead to the loss of valuable time and consequently lives, therefore this English-Croatian dictionary is created in very practical time-saving and easy-to-understand way for both medical professionals and their patients. Instead of one classical A to Z alphabetical order, it consists of over 3000 medical terms divided to several topics where terms regarding each topic are organized alphabetically. The topics start from very basic subjects of numbers and orientation and proceed with terminology concerning accidents and disasters, parts of the human body, injuries, symptoms and diseases, pharmacy, medical facilities, medical procedures, diagnostics, pregnancy and obstetrics.

Ovaj englesko-hrvatski rječnik sadrži preko 3000 medicinskih pojmova prikazanih na jednostavan i razumljiv način koji obuhvaća orijentaciju u prostoru i vremenu; nesreće, katastrofe i pogibeljne situacije; dijelove ljudskog tijela; ozljede, simptome i bolesti; ljekarništvo; medicinske ustanove, njegu i postupke; dijagnostiku, te trudnoću i porodništvo.

CONTENTS - SADRŽAJ

DICTIONARY OF MEDICAL EMERGENCIES
English - Croatian

RJEČNIK HITNIH MEDICINSKIH INTERVENCIJA
Englesko – Hrvatski

NUMBERS	BROJEVI
Zero	Nula
One	Jedan
Two	Dva
Three	Tri
Four	Četiri
Five	Pet
Six	Šest
Seven	Sedam
Eight	Osam
Nine	Devet
Ten	Deset
Eleven	Jedanaest
Twelve	Dvanaest
Thirteen	Trinaest
Fourteen	Četrnaest
Fifteen	Petnaest
Sixteen	Šesnaest
Seventeen	Sedamnaest
Eighteen	Osamnaest
Nineteen	Devetnaest
Twenty	Dvadeset
Twenty-one	Dvadest i jedan
Twenty-two	Dvadeset i dva
Thirty	Trideset
Forty	Četrdeset
Fifty	Pedeset
Sixty	Šezdeset
Seventy	Sedamdeset
Eighty	Osamdeset
Ninety	Devedeset
Hundred	Sto
One hundred and one	Sto jedan
One hundred and twenty-three	Sto dvadeset i tri
Twohundred	Dvjesto
Three hundred	Tristo
Four hundred	Četristo
Five hundred	Petsto
Six hundred	Šesto
Seven hundred	Sedamsto
Eight hundred	Osamsto
Nine hundred	Devetsto
Thousand	Tisuća
Two thousand	Dvije tisuće
Million	Milijun
Milliard (billion)	Milijarda

ORIENTATION IN TIME	ORIJENTACIJA U VREMENU
Yesterday	Jučer
Today	Danas
Tomorrow	Sutra
Year	Godina
Month	Mjesec
Week	Tjedan
Day	Dan
Hour	Sat

Minute	Minuta
Second	Sekunda
Morning	Jutro (prijepodne)
Afternoon	Poslijepodne
Evening	Večer
Night	Noć

ORIENTATION IN SPACE	ORIJENTACIJA U PROSTORU
Up (above)	Gore (iznad)
Down (below)	Dolje (ispod)
Left	Lijevo
Right	Desno
In front	Ispred
Behind	Iza
Inside	Unutra
Outside	Vani

ACCIDENTS, CATASTROPHES AND DISTRESS	NESREĆE, KATASTROFE I POGIBELJNE SITUACIJE
ABC weapons	Atomsko biološko i kemijsko oružje
Air attack	Zračni napad
Airplane crash	Pad aviona
Alarm	Uzbuna
Alarm signal	Znak za uzbunu
Atomic bomb (A-bomb)	Atomska bomba
Atomic weapons	Atomsko oružje
Attack	Napad
Avalanche	Lavina
Bacteria	Bakterija
Biological weapon	Biološko oružje
Bomb	Bomba
Bullet	Metak
Call for help	Poziv u pomoć
Car accident	Automobilska nesreća
Cave	Špilja
Chemical pollution	Kemijsko zagađenje
Chemical weapon	Kemijsko oružje
Civil defense	Civilna zaštita
Cobalt bomb	Kobaltna bomba
Cold weapon	Hladno oružje
Collision	Sudar
Conventional weapon	Konvencionalno oružje
Dirty bomb	Prljava bomba
Domestic accident	Nesreća u kući
Drowned person	Utopljenik
Drowning	Utapanje
Earthquake	Potres
Electric shock	Strujni udar
Enriched uranium	Obogaćeni uranij
Epidemic	Epidemija
Explosion	Eksplozija
Explosive	Eksploziv
Fall	Pad

Fight	Tučnjava
Fire	Vatra
Fire (conflagration)	Požar
Firearm	Vatreno oružje
Flood	Poplava
Heat stroke	Toplotni udar
Helicopter (chopper)	Helikopter
"Help!"	"U pomoć!"
Hidrogen bomb (H-bomb)	Hidrogenska bomba
Homicide (murder)	Ubojstvo
Hostage	Taoc (talac)
Human trafficking	Trgovina ljudima
Hurricane	Uragan
Ice	Led
Iceberg	Ledenjak
Icebreaker	Ledolomac
Invasion	Invazija
Kidnapping	Otmica
Lake	Jezero
Land	Kopno
Land mine	Kopnena mina
Laser weapon	Lasersko oružje
Lava	Lava
Lifebelt (lifebuoy)	Pojas za spašavanje
Lifeboat	Čamac za spašavanje
Lifejacket (life vest)	Prsluk za spašavanje
Marine salvage	Spašavanje broda
Mine	Mina
Mine clearance (demining)	Razminiranje
Mine field	Minsko polje
Mountain	Planina
Naval mine	Morska mina
Neurotoxin	Živčani otrov (neurotoksin)
Neutron bomb	Neutronska bomba
Nuclear accident	Nuklearna nesreća
Nuclear waste (radioactive waste)	Nuklearni otpad (radioaktivni otpad)
Nuclear weapon	Nuklearno oružje
Nuclear weapons testing	Nuklearni pokus
Occupational accident	Nesreća na radu
Pandemic	Pandemija
Parachute	Padobran
Physical assault	Tjelesni napad
Pirate	Gusar
Pirate attack	Gusarski napad
Plutonium	Plutonij
Poison gas	Bojni otrov (otrovni plin)
Radiation	Zračenje
Rape (violation)	Silovanje
Refugee	Izbjeglica
Refugee camp	Izbjeglički logor
Rescuer	Spasilac
River	Rijeka
Robbery	Pljačka
Rock	Stijena
Rope	Uže
Ruins	Ruševine
Salvage	Spašavanje
Sand storm	Pješćana oluja
Sea	More
Sea ice	Santa leda
Search	Potraga
Search and rescue dog	Pas za traganje i spašavanje
Search and rescue team	Ekipa za traganje i spašavanje
Shark attack	Napad morskog psa
Shelter	Sklonište
Ship	Brod
Ship wreck	Olupina broda
Shrapnel	Šrapnel
Sinking of a ship	Potonuće broda
Slavery	Ropstvo
Snow	Snijeg
Snow storm	Snježna mećava
SOS call	SOS poziv
Storm	Nevrijeme (oluja)
Stranding of a ship	Nasukavanje broda
Strategic nuclear weapon	Strateško nuklearno oružje
Stroke (hit, blow)	Udarac
Suicide	Samoubojstvo
Tactical nuclear weapon	Taktičko nuklearno oružje
Terrorist	Terorist
Terrorist attack	Teroristički napad
Terrorist cell	Teroristička ćelija
Thunderclap	Udar groma
Tidal wave	Plimni val
Traffic accident	Prometna nesreća
Tsunami	Tsunami
Typhoon	Tajfun
Uranium	Uranij
Victim	Žrtva
Virus	Virus
Volcanic eruption	Erupcija vulkana
War	Rat
Water	Voda
Waterspout	Morska pijavica
Weapon	Oružje
Weapon of mass destruction	Oružje za masovno uništavanje

PARTS OF THE HUMAN BODY — DIJELOVI LJUDSKOG TIJELA

Abdominal aorta	Abdominalna aorta
Abdominal oblique muscle	Kosi trbušni mišić
Abdominal wall	Trbušna stijenka
Acetabulum	Čašica zdjelične kosti (acetabulum)
Acetylcholine	Acetilkolin
Acoustic nerve (vestibulocochlear nerve)	Slušni živac

Adam's apple	Adamova jabučica	Brain	Mozak
Adductor muscle	Mišić primicač	Brain marrow	Moždana srž
Adenohypophysis	Adenohipofiza	Brain stem	Moždano stablo
Adrenal gland	Nadbubrežna	Brain ventricle	Moždana klijetka
	žlijezda	Breast	Dojka
Adrenalin	Adrenalin	Breastbone	Prsna kost (sternum)
(adrenaline)		(sternum)	
Agglutinin	Aglutinin	Bronchiole	Bronhiola
Agglutinogen	Aglutinogen	Bronchus	Dušnica (bronh)
Albumin	Albumin	Bulbourethral	Bulbouretralna
Aldosterone	Aldosteron	gland (Cowper's	žljezda (Cowperova
Alveolus	Alveola	gland)	žlijezda)
Amino acid	Aminokiselina	Bundle of His	Hisov snopić
Ammonia	Amonijak	Calcaneus	Petna kost
Ankle joint	Skočni zglob		(kalkaneus)
	(gležanj)	Calcitonin	Kalcitonin
Antidiuretic	Antidiuretski	Calf	List
hormone	hormon (vazopresin)	Canal of Schlemm	Schlemmov kanal
(vasopressin)		Canine tooth	Očnjak (kanin)
Anus	Čmar (anus)	Capillary	Kapilara
Anvil (incus)	Nakovanj	Carbohydrate	Ugljikohidrat
Aorta	Aorta	Cardiac atrium	Srčana pretklijetka
Aortic valve	Polumjesečasti		(atrij)
	aortni zalistak	Cardiac muscle	Srčani mišić
Aponeurosis	Široka plosnata	(myocardium)	(miokard)
	tetiva (aponeuroza)	Cardiac ventricle	Srčana klijetka
Arachnoid mater	Paučinasta ovojnica	Carpus	Zapešće
	(arachnoidea)	Cartilage	Hrskavica
Arm	Ruka	Cartilage ring	Hrskavični prsten
Armpit (axilla,	Pazuh (aksila)	Catecholamine	Katekolamin
underarm)		Cell	Stanica
Arteriole	Arteriola	Cementum	Zubni cement
Artery	Arterija	Cerebellum	Mali mozak
Articular capsule	Zglobna čahura	Cerebral cortex	Moždana kora
(joint capsule)		Cerebrospinal fluid	Moždana tekućina
Astrocyte	Astrocit		(likvor)
Atrioventricular	Atrioventrikularni	Cerebrum	Veliki mozak
node	čvor	(telencephalon)	(telencefalon)
Auditory canal (ear	Slušni kanal	Cheek	Obraz
canal)		Chest	Grudište (prsa)
Back	Leđa	Chin	Brada
Bartholin's gland	Bartolinova žlijezda	Cholesterol	Kolesterol
Basophil	Bazofilni granulocit	Choroid	Žilnica
granulocyte		Ciliary muscle	Cilijarni mišić
Belly (abdomen)	Trbuh (abdomen)	Clitoris	Dražica (klitoris)
Biceps brachii	Dvoglavi mišić	Coccygeal vertebra	Trtični kralježak
muscle	nadlaktice	Cochlea	Pužnica
Biceps femoris	Dvoglavi bedreni	Collagen	Kolagen
muscle	mišić	Collarbone	Ključna kost
Bile duct	Žučovod	(clavicle)	(klavikula)
Bilirubin	Bilirubin	Cornea	Rožnica
Blood	Krv	Coronary artery	Koronarna arterija
Blood group	Krvna grupa	Corpus luteum	Žuto tijelo
Blood group A	Krvna grupa A	Corticosteroid	Kortikosteroid
Blood group AB	Krvna grupa AB	Corticosterone	Kortikosteron
Blood group B	Krvna grupa B	Corticotropin	Kortikotropin
Blood group 0	Krvna grupa 0	(adrenocorti-	
Blood vessel	Krvna žila	cotropic hormone)	
Body fluid	Tjelesna tekućina	Cortisol	Kortizol
Bone	Kost	Cortisone	Kortizon
Bone marrow	Koštana srž	Cranial nerve	Moždani živac
Brachialis muscle	Nadlaktični mišić	Crown ofa tooth	Kruna zuba

Deltoid muscle	Rameni mišić (deltoideus)	Globulin	Globulin
Dendrite	Dendrit	Glomerulus	Glomerul
Dental pulp	Središte zuba (pulpa)	Glucagon	Glukagon
Dentin	Zubni dentin	Glucocorticoid	Glukokortikoid
Deoxyribonucleic acid (DNA)	Dezoksiribonukleins ka kiselina (DNK)	Glucose	Glukoza
Diaphragm	Ošit (dijafragma)	Gluteal muscle	Sjedni mišić
Diencephalon	Međumozak	Glycogen	Glikogen
Duodenum	Dvanaesnik (duodenum)	Gonadotrophin	Gonadotropin
Dura mater	Tvrda moždana ovojnica	Granulocyte	Granulocit
Ear	Uho	Groin	Prepona
Eardrum (tympanic membrane)	Bubnjić	Growth hormone (somatotrophin)	Hormon rasta (somatotropin)
Earwax (cerumen)	Ušna mast (ušna smola, cerumen)	Gullet (oesophagus)	Jednjak
Ejaculatory duct	Sjemenovod	Gums (gingiva)	Desni
Elastin	Elastin	Hair	Dlaka
Elbow	Lakat	Hair	Kosa
Elbow joint	Lakatni zglob	Hammer (malleus)	Čekić (malleus)
Electrolyte	Elektrolit	Hand	Šaka
Eosinophil	Eozinofil	Hard palate	Tvrdo nepce
Epididymis	Pasjemenik	Head	Glava
Erythrocyte (red blood cell)	Eritrocit (crveno krvno tjelešce)	Heart	Srce
Estradiol	Folikulin (estradiol)	Heart valve (cardiac valve)	Srčani zalistak
Estrogen	Estrogen	Heel	Peta
Ethmoid bone	Sitasta kost (etmoidna kost)	Hemoglobin	Hemoglobin
Eye	Oko	Hip bone	Kost kuka
Eye orbit	Očna šupljina	Hip joint	Kuk (zglob kuka)
Eyeball	Očna jabučica	Hormone	Hormon
Eyebrow	Obrva	Hymen	Djevičnjak (himen)
Eyelash	Trepavica	Hyoid bone (lingual bone)	Podjezična kost
Eyelid	Kapak	Hypophysis (pituitary gland)	Hipofiza
Face	Lice	Hypothalamus	Hipotalamus
Fallopian tube (oviduct)	Jajovod	Ileum	Ileum
Fat	Mast	Ilium	Crijevna kost
Fat tissue	Masno tkivo	Immunoglobulin	Imunoglobulin
Fibrin	Fibrin	Incisor	Sjekutić (inciziv)
Fibrinogen	Fibrinogen	Inferior vena cava	Donja šuplja vena
Fibroblast	Fibroblast	Innominate bone (pelvis)	Zdjelica
Fibula (calf bone)	Lisna kost (fibula)	Insulin	Inzulin
Finger	Ručni prst	Intercostal muscle	Međurebreni mišić
Foot	Stopalo	Interstitial fluid	Međustanična tekućina
Forearm	Podlaktica	Intervertebral disc	Međukralježnični disk
Forefinger	Kažiprst	Intestinal juice	Crijevni sok
Forehead	Čelo	Intestinal villus	Crijevna resica
Foreskin (prepuce)	Prepucij	Intestine	Crijevo
Frontal bone	Čeona kost	Iris	Šarenica
Gall (bile)	Žuč	Ischium	Sjedna kost
Gall bladder	Žućni mjehur	Jaw	Čeljust
Gas	Plin	Jejunum	Jejunum
Gastric acid	Želučana kiselina	Joint	Zglob
Gastric juice	Želučani sok	Joint cartilage	Zglobna hrskavica
Gastric mucous membrane	Želučana sluznica	Keratin	Keratin
		Kidney	Bubreg
Gland	Žlijezda	Knee	Koljeno
Glans	Glavić	Kneecap (patella)	Iver (patela)
		Lachrymal bone	Suzna kost
		Lachrymal gland	Suzna žlijezda

Large intestine (colon)	Debelo crijevo	Neck	Vrat
Larynx	Grkljan	Nerve	Živac
Leg	Noga	Nipple	Bradavica
Lens	Leća	Noradrenaline	Noradrenalin
Leukocyte	Leukocit	Nose	Nos
Ligament	Ligament	Nostril	Nosnica
Lip	Usna	Occipital bone	Zatiljna kost
Little finger (pinky)	Mali prst	Optic nerve	Vidni živac
Liver	Jetra	Organ	Organ
Loin	Križa	Ovary	Jajnik
Lower jaw (mandible)	Donja čeljust (mandibula)	Ovum	Jajašce
		Oxytocin	Oksitocin
Lower leg	Potkoljenica	Palate	Nepce
Lumbar vertebra	Slabinski kralježak (lumbalni kralježak)	Palatine bone	Nepčana kost
		Palm	Dlan
Lung	Plućno krilo	Pancreas	Gušterača
Lungs	Pluća	Pancreatic juice	Sok gušterače
Luteinising hormone	Luteinizirajući hormon	Parasympathetic nervous system	Parasimpatikus
Lymph	Limfa	Parathyroid gland	Doštitnjača
Lymph gland (lymph node)	Limfna žlijezda	Parathyroid hormone	Paratireoidni hormon
Lymph vessel	Limfna žila	Parietal bone	Tjemena kost
Lymphocyte	Limfocit	Parietal pleura	Porebrica (parijetalna pleura)
Masseter muscle	Žvakaći mišić		
Medulla oblongata	Produžena moždina	Pectoralis major muscle	Veliki prsni mišić
Melanin	Melanin		
Melanotropin	Melanotropin	Pectoralis minor muscle	Mali prsni mišić
Melatonin	Melatonin		
Meninx	Moždana ovojnica	Penis	Penis
Meniscus	Zglobni menisk	Pericardium	Osrčje (perikard)
Metacarpal bone	Kost pesti (metakarpalna kost)	Perineum	Međica (perineum)
		Peritoneum	Potrbušnica (peritoneum)
Metacarpus	Pest (metakarpus)		
Metatarsal bone	Kost donožja (metatarzalna kost)	Phalanx bone	Kost prsta (falanga)
		Pharynx (gullet, gorge)	Ždrijelo
Metatarsus	Donožje (metatarzus)	Phospholipid	Fosfolipid
		Pia mater	Meka moždana ovojnica
Middle ear	Srednje uho		
Middle finger	Srednji prst	Pineal body (pineal gland, epiphysis)	Pinealna žlijezda (epifiza)
Milk tooth	Mliječni zub		
Mineralcorticoid	Mineralkortikoid (Na-hormon)	Pinna (auricle)	Ušna školjka
		Plasma	Plazma
Mitral valve (bicuspid valve)	Mitralni zalistak (bikuspidalni zalistak)	Pleura	Pleura
		Pore	Pora
		Portal vein	Portalna vena
Molar	Kutnjak (molar)	Premolar	Pretkutnjak (premolar)
Monocyte	Monocit		
Mouth	Usta	Progesterone	Progesteron
Mouth cavity (oral cavity)	Usna šupljina	Prostate	Prostata
		Protein	Bjelančevina (protein)
Mucous membrane	Sluznica		
Mucus	Sluz	Pubis (pubic bone)	Stidna kost
Muscle	Mišić	Pulmonary artery	Plućna arterija
Muscular fascia	Mišićna fascija	Pupil	Zjenica
Nail	Nokat	Quadriceps femoris muscle	Četveroglavi bedreni mišić
Nape (occiput)	Zatiljak		
Nasal bone	Nosna kost	Radius	Palčana kost
Nasolacrimal duct (tear duct)	Suzno-nosni kanal	Rectus abdominis muscle	Ravni trbušni mišić
Navel (belly button)	Pupak	Retina	Mrežnica (retina)

Rh factor negative	Negativan Rh faktor	Sympathetic nervous system	Simpatikus
Rh factor positive	Pozitivan Rh faktor		
Rhomboid muscle	Romboidni mišić	Synapse	Sinapsa
Rib	Rebro	Synovial bursa	Sluzna vreća (bursa)
Rib cage	Grudni koš	Synovial fluid (synovia)	Zglobna tekućina (sinovijalna tekućina)
Ribonucleic acid	Ribonukleinska kiselina		
Ring finger	Prstenjak	Synovial membrane	Sinovijalna opna
Root of a tooth	Korijen zuba	Tailbone (coccyx)	Trtica
Sacral vertebra	Krstačni kralježak (sakralni kralježak)	Tailor's muscle (sartorius muscle)	Krojački mišić
Saliva (spit, slobber)	Slina (pljuvačka)	Tarsal bone	Kost zastoplja (kost tarzusa)
Salivary gland	Žlijezda slinovnica	Tarsus	Zastoplje
Scalp	Vlasište	Taste bud	Okusni pupoljak
Sclera	Bjeloočnica	Tear	Suza
Sebaceous gland	Žlijezda lojnica	Temple	Sljepoočnica
Sebum	Loj	Temporal bone	Sljepoočna kost
Semen	Sperma	Tendon (sinew)	Tetiva
Semimembranosus muscle	Poluopnasti mišić	Testicle	Jaje (mudo, testis)
		Testosterone	Testosteron
Seminal vesicle	Sjemena vrećica	Thalamus	Talamus
Semitendinosus muscle	Polutetivni mišić	Thigh	Natkoljenica (bedro)
		Thighbone (femur)	Bedrena kost (femur)
Sesamoid bone	Sezamska kost	Thoracic aorta	Torakalna aorta
Sex gland (gonad)	Spolna žlijezda	Thoracic vertebra	Leđni kralježak (grudni ili torakalni kralježak)
Shinbone (tibia)	Goljenica (tibija)		
Shoulder	Rame		
Shoulder blade (scapula)	Lopatica (skapula)	Throat	Grlo
		Thrombocyte	Trombocit
Shoulder joint	Rameni zglob	Thumb	Palac
Sigmoid colon	Sigmoidni dio debelog crijeva	Thymus	Grudna žlijezda (timus)
Sinus	Sinus	Thyroid	Štitnjača
Skeleton	Kostur	Thyroid-stimulating hormone (TSH, thyrotropin)	Tireotropin (TSH)
Skin	Koža		
Skull	Lubanja		
Skull base	Baza lubanje	Thyroxine	Tiroksin
Small intestine	Tanko crijevo	Tissue	Tkivo
Smooth muscle	Glatki mišić	Toe	Nožni prst
Soft palate	Meko nepce	Tongue	Jezik
Sole	Taban	Tonsil	Krajnik
Sperm (spermatozoon)	Spermij	Tooth	Zub
		Tooth enamel	Zubna caklina
Sphenoid bone	Klinasta kost (leptirasta kost)	Trapezius muscle	Trapezni mišić
		Triceps brachii muscle	Troglavi mišić nadlaktice
Sphincter	Kružni mišić (sfinkter)		
		Triceps surae muscle	Troglavi mišić potkoljenice
Spinal cord	Kralježnična moždina		
		Tricuspid valve	Trolisni zalistak
Spinal nerve	Spinalni živac	Triglyceride	Triglicerid
Spine (spinal column, backbone)	Kralježnica	Triiodothyronine	Trijodtironin
		Trunk (torso)	Trup (torzo)
Spleen	Slezena	Tympanic cavity	Bubnjište
Stirrup (stapes)	Stremen	Ulna	Lakatna kost (ulna)
Stomach	Želudac	Upper arm	Nadlaktica
Stool (feces)	Stolica (feces, izmet)	Upper arm bone (humerus)	Nadlaktična kost (humerus)
Striated muscle	Poprečno-prugasti mišić		
		Upper back	Gornji dio leđa
Superior vena cava	Gornja šuplja vena	Upper jaw (maxilla)	Gornja čeljust (maksila)
Sweat	Znoj		
Sweat gland	Žlijezda znojnica		

Urea	Mokraćevina (urea, ureja)	Abrasion	Ojedina (abrazija)
Ureter	Mokraćovod (ureter)	Abscess	Apsces
Urethra	Vanjska mokraćna cijev (uretra)	Absence in development of an organ (aplasia of an organ)	Nerazvijenost organa (aplazija organa)
Urinary bladder	Mokraćni mjehur		
Urine	Mokraća (urin)	Absence of menstrual period (amenorrhea)	Izostanak mjesečnice (amenoreja)
Vagina	Rodnica (vagina)		
Valve (valvula)	Zalistak		
Vein	Vena	Absence of pulse	Gubitak pulsa
Ventricle	Klijetka	Acariasis	Akarijaza
Venule	Venula	Accelerated basal metabolism	Ubrzan bazalni metabolizam
Vermiform appendix (cecal appaendix)	Slijepo crijevo (crvuljak)		
		Accelerated pulse rate	Ubrzani puls
Vertebra	Kralježak	Achilles tendon overuse injury	Sindrom prenaprezanja Ahilove tetive
Vertex (crown of head)	Tjeme		
Vestibule	Predvorje (vestibulum)	Achilles tendon rupture	Puknuće Ahilove tetive
Visceral pleura	Poplućnica (visceralna pleura)	Achillodynia (Achilles tendinitis)	Ahilodinija (tendinitis Ahilove tetive)
Vocal chord	Glasnica		
Vomer	Raonik (vomer)	Achlorhydria	Aklorhidrija
Vulva	Stidnica	Achondroplasia	Ahondroplazija
Windpipe (trachea)	Dušnik	Acidosis	Acidoza
Womb (uterus)	Maternica (uterus)	Acne	Akne
Wrist	Ručni zglob	Acne vulgaris	Vulgarne akne
Wrist bone (carpal bone)	Kost zapešća (karpalna kost)	Acoustic neuroma	Neurom slušnog živca
Zygoma (cheekbone, malar bone)	Sponična kost	Acrocyanosis	Akrocijanoza
		Acromegaly	Akromegalija
		Acrophobia (fear of heights)	Akrofobija (strah od visine)
SYMPTOMS, INJURIES AND DISEASES	SIMPTOMI, OZLJEDE I BOLESTI	Actinic keratosis	Aktinička keratoza
		Actinomycosis	Aktinomikoza
		Acute abdomen	Akutni abdomen
		Acute appendicitis	Akutna upala crvuljka
Abdominal aortic aneurysm	Aneurizma abdominalne aorte		
		Acute gastric dilatation	Akutna dilatacija želuca
Abdominal colic	Trbušna kolika (abdominalna kolika)		
		Acute kidney failure	Akutno zatajenje bubrega
Abdominal pain	Bol u trbuhu		
Abdominal wall tension	Napetost trbušne stijenke	Acute lymphoblastic leukemia	Akutna limfatična leukemija
Aberrant pancreas	Aberantni pankreas	Acute myeloid leukemia (AML)	Akutna mijeloična leukemija
Abnormal flexibility	Abnormalna gibljivost		
		Acute pain	Akutna bol
Abnormal twisting of the intestines (volvulus)	Zapletaj crijeva	Acute pulmonary heart	Akutno plućno srce
		Addiction	Ovisnost
Abnormally heavy menstrual period (menorrhagia)	Abnormalno velik gubitak krvi tijekom mjesečnice (menoragija)	Addison's disease	Addisonova bolest
		Adenocarcinoma	Adenokarcinom
		Adenoma	Adenom
		Adenopathy	Adenopatija
Abnormally large intake of food (hyperphagia)	Prekomjerno jedenje (hiperfagija)	African trypanosomiasis (sleeping sickness)	Afrička tripanosomijaza (bolest spavanja)
Aboulia (disorder of diminished motivation)	Abulija (poremećaj umanjene motivacije)	Age-related hearing loss (presbycusis)	Staračka nagluhost (prezbiakuzija)

Age-related long-sightedness (presbyopia)	Staračka dalekovidnost (prezbiopija)	Anemia	Slabokrvnost (anemija)
Agenesis (absence of an organ)	Agenezija (nedostatak jednog organa)	Anemia of chronic disease	Anemija kronične bolesti
		Anencephaly	Anencefalija
Agnail (hangnail)	Zanoktica	Aneurysm (aneurism)	Aneurizma
Agranulocytosis	Agranulocitoza	Aneurysm rupture	Prsnuće aneurizme
AIDS (acquired immune deficiency syndrome)	SIDA (sindrom stečene imunodeficijencije, AIDS)	Angina	Angina
		Angina pectoris	Angina pektoris
		Angioedema (angioneurotic edema)	Angioedem (Quinckeov edem, angioneurotski edem)
Air embolism (gas embolism)	Zračna embolija		
Albinism	Albinizam	Angioma	Angiom
Albuminuria	Albuminurija	Angiosarcoma	Angiosarkom
Alcohol poisoning	Trovanje alkoholom	Anisakiasis	Anisakijaza
Alcoholic cardiomyopathy	Alkoholna kardiomiopatja	Ankle arthrosis	Artroza skočnog zgloba
Alcoholic cirrhosis	Alkoholna ciroza	Ankle distortion	Uganuće skočnog zgloba
Alcoholism	Alkoholizam		
Aldosteronism (hyperaldosteronism)	Aldosteronizam	Ankle impingement syndrome	Prednji sindrom sraza gornjeg nožnog zgloba
Algodystrophy	Algodistrofija		
Alkali poisoning	Trovanje alkalima	Ankylosing spondylitis (Bechterew's syndrome)	Ankilozantni spondilitis (Bechterewov sindrom)
Alkalosis	Alkaloza		
Allergic contact dermatitis	Alergijski kontaktni dermatitis		
		Ankylosis (joint stiffness)	Ankiloza (ukočenje zgloba)
Allergic conjunctivitis	Alergijski konjuktivitis	Anorexia	Anoreksija
Allergic rhinitis	Alergijski rinitis	Ant sting	Ugriz mrava
Allergy	Alergija	Anterior cruciate ligament rupture (ACL rupture)	Razdor prednje ukrižene sveze koljenskog zgloba
Alopecia	Ćelavost		
Alopecia areata	Alopecia areata		
Alopecia universalis	Opća alopecija	Anthracosis	Antrakoza
Altitude sickness (acute mountain sickness)	Visinska bolest	Anthrax	Antraks (bedrenica, crni prišt)
		Anuria (passage of urine < 100 ml in 24 hours)	Anurija (lučenje urina < 100 ml u 24 sata)
Alzheimer's diesase	Alzheimerova bolest		
Amebiasis (amebic dysentery)	Amebijaza		
Amnesia	Amnezija	Anxiety	Nemir (anksioznost)
Amputation	Amputacija	Aortic aneurysm	Aneurizma aorte
Amyloidosis	Amiloidoza	Aortic dissection	Disekcija aorte
Amyotrophic lateral sclerosis	Amiotrofična lateralna skleroza	Aortic valve stenosis	Stenoza aortnog ušća
Anal abscess	Analni apsces	Aortoiliac occlusive disease (Leriche's syndrome)	Lericheov sindrom
Anal atresia	Atrezija anusa		
Anal bleeding	Krvarenje iz analnog otvora		
		Aphtha (mouth ulcer)	Afte (ulceracija sluznice usta)
Anal fissure	Analna fisura	Aplasia	Aplazija
Anal fistula	Analna fistula	Aplastic anemia	Aplastična anemija
Analgesia (loss of pain sensation)	Analgezija (neosjetljivost na bol)	Apoplexy	Moždano krvarenje (apopleksija)
Anaphylactic shock	Anafilaktični šok	Appetite	Apetit
Anaplastic carcinoma	Anaplastični karcinom	Appetite changes	Promjene apetita
		Aquaphobia	Hidrofobija
Ancylostomiasis	Ankilostomijaza	Arrhythmia	Aritmija
Androblastoma (Sertoli-Leydig cell tumor)	Androblastom (tumor Sertoli-Leydigovih stanica)	Arrhytmogenic right ventricular dysplasia	Aritmogena displazija desne klijetke

Arsenic poisoning	Trovanje arsenom	Bacteriuria	Bakteriurija
Arterial bleeding	Arterijsko krvarenje	Bad breath	Zadah iz usta
Arterial embolism	Arterijska embolija	(halitosis)	(halitoza)
Arteriosclerosis	Arterioskleroza	Balance disorder	Poremećaj ravnoteže
Arthrogryposis	Artrogripoza	Ball-shaped	Kuglasta aneurizma
Arthropathy	Artropatija	aneurysm of the	arterije mozga
Arthrosis	Artroza	brain artery	
(osteoarthritis,	(osteoartritis,	Barotrauma	Barotrauma
degenerative	degenerativni	Bartonellosis	Bartoneloza
arthritis)	artritis)	Basal cell	Karcinom bazalnih
Asbestos poisoning	Trovanje azbestom	carcinoma	stanica (bazaliom)
Asbestosis	Azbestoza	Base of skull	Prijelom baze
Ascaridosis	Askaridijaza	fracture (basal skull	lubanje
Ascites	Ascites	fracture)	
Aspergilloma	Aspergilom	Basedow Graves	Basedowljeva bolest
(mycetoma, fungus		disease	
ball)		Basophilia	Bazofilija
Aspergillosis	Aspergiloza	Bedsore (decubitus	Dekubitus
Asphyxia	Asfiksija	ulcer)	
Asthma	Astma	Behavioral disorder	Poremećaj ponašanja
Astigmatism	Astigmatizam	Behçet's disease	Behçetova bolest
Astrocytoma	Astrocitom	Bell's palsy	Bellova paraliza
Atherosclerosis	Ateroskleroza	Bell's phenomenon	Bellov fenomen
Athetosis	Atetoza	Benign positional	Benigna pozicijska
Athlete's foot (tinea	Atletsko stopalo	vertigo	vrtoglavica
pedis)	(gljivična infekcija	Benign prostatic	Benigna hipertrofija
	stopala, tinea pedis)	hyperthroph	prostate
Athlete's heart	Sportsko srce	Benign tumor	Dobroćudni tumor
(cardiac			(benigni tumor)
hypertrophy)		Bile duct atresia	Atrezija žučnih
Atony (atonia)	Atonija		vodova
Atopic dermatitis	Atopijski dermatitis	Biliary cirrhosis	Bilijarna ciroza
Atrial fibrillation	Atrijska fibrilacija	Biliary colic	Žučna kolika
Atrial septal defect	Atrijski septalni	Biot's respiration	Biotovo disanje
	defekt	Bipolar disorder	Bipolarni poremećaj
Atrioventricular	Atrijskoventrikularni	(manic-depressive	(manično-depresivna
block (AV block)	blok	psychosis)	psihoza)
Atrophy	Atrofija	Bird flu (influenza	Ptičja gripa podtip
Attention deficit	Poremećaj	virus A subtype	H5N1
disorder	koncentracije	H5N1)	
Atypical pneumonia	Atipična upala pluća	Birthmark (nevus)	Madež (nevus)
Autism	Autizam	Bite	Ugriz
Autoimmune	Autoimunološka	Bite by rabies	Ugriz bijesne
disease	bolest	infected animal	životinje
Aviophobia (fear of	Aerofobija (strah od	Bite wound	Ugrizna rana
flying)	letenja)	Black stool (melena)	Crna stolica
Avitaminosis	Avitamonoza		(melena)
Baby colic	Novorođenačke	Black widow bite	Ugriz crne udovice
	kolike	Bladder stone	Kamenac mokraćnog
Back pain	Bol u leđima	(urolithiasis)	mjehura
(dorsalgia)	(dorzopatija)	Blast-syndrome	Blast-sindrom
Bacteremia	Bakterijemija	Blastoma	Blastom
Bacterial	Bakterijski	Blastomycosis	Blastomikoza
conjunctivitis	konjuktivitis	Bleeding	Krvarenje
Bacterial	Bakterijski	(haemorrhage)	(hemoragija)
endocarditis	endokarditis	Bleeding into joint	Krvarenje u zglob
Bacterial infection	Bakterijska infekcija	space	(hemartroza)
Bacterial	Bakterijska upala	(hemarthrosis)	
pneumonia	pluća	Bleeding into the	Krvarenje u jajovod
Bacterial vaginosis	Bakterijska infekcija	fallopian tube	(hematosalpinks)
	rodnice (bakterijska	(hematosalpinx)	
	vaginoza)	Blepharitis	Blefaritis

Blindness	Sljepoća	Broken bone (bone	Prijelom kosti
Blister	Plik	fracture)	(fraktura kosti)
Blister (corn)	Žulj (plik, kurje oko)	Broken collar bone	Prijelom ključne
Bloating and gases	Nadutost i vjetrovi	(clavicle fracture)	kosti
(flatulence)		Broken elbow	Prijelom lakatnog
Blood clot	Krvni ugrušak	(olecranon	vrha (prijelom
(thrombus)	(tromb)	fracture)	olekranona)
Blood in	Krv u likvoru	Broken fibula	Prijelom lisne kosti
cerebrospinal fluid		(fibula fracture)	
Blood in sputum	Krvavi iskašljaj	Broken finger	Prijelom članka prsta
(hemoptysis)	(hemoptiza)	(finger fracture)	
Blood in stool	Krv u stolici	Broken foot	Prijelom kosti
(hematochezia)	(hematohezija)	(metatarsal	stopala
Blood in urine	Krv u urinu	fracture)	
(hematuria)	(hematurija)	Broken forearm	Prijelom obje
Blood pressure fall	Pad krvnog tlaka	(fractured ulna and	podlaktične kosti
Blood vessel	Bolesti krvnih žila	radius)	
diseases		Broken heel bone	Prijelom petne kosti
Blount's disease	Blountova bolest	(calcaneus fracture)	
Bone bending (bone	Savijanje kosti	Broken knee cap	Prijelom ivera
torsion)		(patellar fracture)	(prijelom patele)
Bone tuberculosis	Tuberkuloza kosti	Broken lower leg	Prijelom obje kosti
Borderline	Granični poremećaj	bones (fractured	potkoljenice
personality disorder	osobnosti	tibia and fibula)	
Bornholm disease	Bornholmska bolest	Broken navicular	Prijelom navikularne
(epidemic myalgia)	(epidemijska	bone (navicular	kosti
	mialgija)	fracture)	
Borreliosis	Borelioza	Broken pelvis	Prijelom zdjelice
Botryoid sarcoma	Botrioidni sarkom	(pelvis fracture)	
Botulism	Botulizam	Broken rib (rib	Prijelom rebra
Bouchard's nodes	Bouchardovi čvorići	fracture)	
Bow legs (genu	Genu varum	Broken shinbone	Prijelom goljenične
varum)		(tibia fracture)	kosti
Bowen's disease	Bowenova bolest	Broken shoulder	Prijelom lopatice
(squamous cell		blade (scapula	
carcinoma in situ)		fracture)	
Brachial syndrome	Brahijalni sindrom	Broken thighbone	Prijelom bedrene
	bolne nadlaktice	(femur fracture)	kosti
Brain abscess	Apsces mozga	Broken ulna (ulna	Prijelom lakatne
Brain compression	Kompresija mozga	fracture)	kosti
Brain concussion	Potres mozga	Broken upper arm	Prijelom nadlaktice
Brain development	Anomalija u razvoju	(humerus fracture)	
anomaly	mozga	Broken vertebral	Prijelom trupa
Brain laceration	Laceracija mozga	body (vertebral	kralješka
Breast cancer	Rak dojke	corpus fracture)	
Breast carcinoma	Karcinom dojke	Bronchial carcinoid	Karcinoid bronha
Breast pain	Bol u dojci	Bronchial	Karcinom bronha
(mastalgia)	(mastalgija)	carcinoma	
Breathing difficulty	Otežano disanje	Bronchiectasis	Bronhiektazije
Breathing sound	Glasno otežano	Bronchopleural	Bronhopleuralna
due to blockage in	disanje (stridor)	fistula	fistula
the airway (stridor)		Bronchopneumonia	Bronhopneumonija
Brenner tumour	Brennerov tumor	Bronchospasm	Bronhospazam
Brill's disease	Brillova bolest	Brown urine	Smeđi urin
	(Brill-Zinsserova	Brucellosis	Bruceloza (malteška
	bolest)		ili sredozemna
Brodie abscess	Brodijev apsces		groznica, Bangova
Broken ankle (ankle	Prijelom gležnja		bolest)
fracture)		Bruise (ecchymosis)	Modrica (ekhimoza)
Broken big toe	Prijelom falange	Buerger's disease	Buergerova bolest
(fractured hallux)	nožnog palca	(thromboangiitis	
		obliterans)	

Bulging eyes (exophthalmos)	Izbuljene oči (egzoftalmus)
Bulimia	Bulimija
Bundle branch block	Blok grane Hisovog snopića
Bunion	Čukalj
Burn	Opeklina
Burning sensation	Pećenje (žarenje)
Burping (belching)	Podrigivanje
Byssinosis (Monday fever)	Bisinoza
Cachexia	Kaheksija
Cadmium poisoning	Trovanje kadmijem
Calcification	Ovapnjenje (kalcifikacija)
Callosity (thickening)	Zadebljanje kože
Candidiasis (thrush)	Kandidijaza
Capillary hemangioma (infantile hemangioma, strawberry hemangioma)	Kapilarni hemangiom
Carbon monoxide poisoning	Trovanje ugljičnim monoksidom
Carbuncle	Karbunkul
Carcinoid	Karcinoid
Carcinoid syndrome	Karcinoidni sindrom
Carcinoma	Karcinom
Carcinosis	Karcinoza
Cardiac arrest (cardiopulmonary arrest)	Zastoj srca (srčani arest)
Cardiac arrhythmia	Srčana aritmija
Cardiac asthma (paroxysmal nocturnal dyspnea)	Srčana astma (paroksizmalna dispneja)
Cardiac decompensation	Srčana dekompenzacija
Cardiogenic shock	Kardiogeni šok
Cardiomyopathy	Kardiomiopatija
Cardiotoxicity	Toksična kardiomiopatija
Carpal tunnel syndrome	Sindrom karpalnog tunela
Cat bite	Ugriz mačke
Cat cry syndrome (5p minus syndrome, Lejeune's syndrome)	Sindrom mačjeg krika
Catalepsy	Katalepsija
Cataplexy	Katapleksija
Cataract	Mrena (katarakta)
Catarrh	Katar
Cavernous hemangioma	Kavernozni hemangiom
Cellulitis	Celulitis
Cephalocele	Cefalokela
Cercaria	Cerkarija
Cerebral aneurysm	Cerebralna aneurizma
Cerebral contusion	Nagnječenje mozga
Cerebral edema	Edem mozga
Cerebral palsy	Cerebralna paraliza
Cerebrovascular anomaly	Anomalija moždanih krvnih žila
Cervical cancer	Rak grlića maternice
Cervical carcinoma	Karcinom grlića maternice
Cervical dysplasia	Cervikalna displazija
Cervical erosion	Cervikalna erozija
Cervical polyp	Polip na grliću maternice
Cervical rib	Vratno rebro
Cervicobrachial syndrome	Sindrom vrat-rame (cervikobrahijalni sindrom)
Cervicocephal syndrome	Cervikocefalni sindrom
Chagas disease (American trypanosomiasis)	Chagasova bolest (americka tripanosomijaza)
Chalicosis	Kalikoza
Chancre	Čankir
Chancroid (soft chancre)	Meki čankir
Changes in consciousness	Promjene stanja svijesti
Changes in moles	Promjene na madežima
Changes in mucous membrane	Promjene na sluznici
Changes in olfactory sensation	Promjene osjeta mirisa
Changes in shape of bones	Promjene oblika kosti
Changes in tactile sensation	Promjene osjeta dodira
Changes in taste sensation	Promjene osjeta okusa
Charcot-Marie-Tooth disease	Bolest Charcot-Marie-Tooth
Chemical conjunctivitis	Kemijski konjuktivitis
Chemical injuries	Kemijske ozljede
Chemical warfare poisoning	Trovanje kemijskim oružjem
Chest pain	Bol u prsištu
Chicken-pox	Vodene kozice (varičela)
Chikungunya	Chikungunya virusna bolest
Chilblain (perniosis)	Smrzotina
Childhood infectious diseases	Dječje zarazne bolesti
Chlamydia infection	Klamidijska infekcija
Choking (suffocation)	Gušenje

Cholangiocellular carcinoma	Kolangiocelularni karcinom
Cholera	Kolera
Chondroblastoma	Hondroblastom
Chondroma	Hondrom
Chondromalacia patellae (runner's knee, patello-femoral pain syndrome)	Hondromalacija patele (trkačko koljeno, sindrom patelofemoralne boli)
Chondromyxoid fibroma	Hondromiksoidni fibrom
Chondrosarcoma	Hondrosarkom
Choreoathetosis	Koreoatetoza
Choriocarcinoma	Koriokarcinom
Chromoblastomy-cosis (chromomycosis, Pedroso's disease)	Kromomikoza
Chronic cerebrospinal venous insufficiency	Kronična cerebrospinalna venozna insuficijencija
Chronic fatigue syndrome	Sindrom kroničnog umora
Chronic lymphocytic leukemia	Kronična limfocitna leukemija
Chronic myeloid leukemia	Kronična mijeloična leukemija
Chronic obstructive pulmonary disease	Kronična opstruktivna plućna bolest
Chronic pain	Kronična bol
Chronic paroxysmal hemicrania (Sjaastad syndrome)	Kronična paroksizmalna hemikranija (Sjaastadov sindrom)
Chronic renal failure	Kronično zatajenje bubrega
Chylothorax	Hilotoraks
Claustrophobia (fear of closed space)	Klaustrofobija (strah od zatvorenog prostora)
Cleft lip and palate	Rascjep usne i nepca
Clonorchiasis	Klonorkijaza
Clostridium perfringens toxic infection	Toksična infekcija Clostridium perfringensom
Club foot (talipes equinovarus)	Čopavo stopalo (uvrnuto stopalo, pes equinovarus)
Cluster headache	Cluster glavobolja
Coagulation factor deficiency	Manjak faktora koagulacije
Coarctation of the aorta	Koarktacija aorte
Coccidioidomycosis (San Joaquin Valley fever)	Kokcidioidomikoza (San Joaquin Valley vrućica)
Coccygodynia	Kokcigodinija
Coeliac disease (celiac disease)	Celijakija
Colic	Kolika
Collapse	Kolaps
Colon diverticulum	Divertikul na debelom crijevu
Colon polyp	Polip na debelom crijevu
Colorado tick fever (mountain tick fever)	Groznica planinskog krpelja
Coma	Koma
Comminuted fracture	Kominutivni prijelom kosti
Common cold	Prehlada (hunjavica)
Compartment syndrome	Sindrom fascijalnog prostora
Confusion	Smetenost
Congenital aneurysm of arteries at the base of the brain	Urođena aneurizma arterija baze mozga
Congenital dysplasia of the hip (congenital hip dislocation)	Urođeno iščašenje kuka (kongenitalna displazija kuka)
Congenital heart defect	Urođena srčana greška
Congenital heart disease (congenital cardiopathy)	Urođena srčana bolest (kongenitalna kardiopatija)
Congenital pyloric stenosis	Urođena stenoza pilorusa
Conjunctival foreign body	Konjuktivitis izazvan stranim tijelom
Constipation (obstipation)	Zatvor (opstipacija)
Contact dermatitis	Kontaktni dermatitis
Contracture	Kontraktura
Contusion	Nagnječenje (zgnječenje, kontuzija)
Convulsions	Konvulzije
Coronary disease	Koronarna bolest (koronaropatija)
Cough	Kašalj
Cradle cap (infantile seborrhoeic dermatitis)	Tjemenica (dojenačka seboreja)
Cranial neuralgia	Neuralgija moždanih živaca
Crepitation	Krepitacija
Creutzfeldt-Jakob disease (so called "mad cow disease")	Creutzfeldt-Jakobova bolest (tzv. "kravlje ludilo")
Crimean-Congo hemorrhagic fever	Krimska hemoragijska groznica
Crohn's disease	Crohnova bolest

Crotch itch (tinea cruris)	Gljivična infekcija prepona (tinea cruris)
Croup (acute obstructive laryngitis)	Krup (akutni opstruktivni laringitis)
Crush-syndrome	Crush-sindrom
Crust (scab)	Krasta
Cryptococcosis	Kriptokokoza
Cryptogenic cirrhosis	Kriptogena ciroza
Cryptorchidism	Retencija testisa (kriptorhizam)
Cushing's syndrome (hypercorticism)	Cushingov sindrom (hiperkortikolizam)
Cut wound	Rezna rana (posjekotina)
Cutaneous leishmaniasis (Oriental sore)	Orijentalni ulkus (kožna lišmenijaza)
Cyanide poisoning	Trovanje cijanidom
Cyanosis	Cijanoza
Cyst	Cista
Cystadenocarcinoma	Cistadenokarcinom
Cystadenofibroma	Cistadenofibrom
Cystadenoma	Cistadenom
Cystic fibrosis	Cistična fibroza
Cysticercosis	Cisticerkoza
Cystoma	Cistom
Daltonism	Daltonizam
Dancer's foot (pes equinus)	Balerinsko stopalo (pes equinus)
Dancer's tendinitis (flexor hallucis tendinitis)	Tendinitis plesača (tendinitis dugog pregibača palca)
Dandruff	Perut
Day blindness (hemeralopia)	Kokošje sljepilo (hemeralopija)
Deafness	Gluhoća
Death	Smrt
Decompression sickness (diver's disease, caisson disease)	Dekompresijska bolest (kesonska bolest)
Decreased body temperature (hypothermia)	Snižena temperatura tijela (hipotermija)
Decreased production of urine (oliguria)	Smanjeno izlučivanje urina (oligurija)
Dehydration	Dehidracija
Delayed puberty	Zakašnjeli pubertet
Delirium	Delirij
Dementia	Demencija
Demineralization	Demineralizacija
Dengue fever	Dengue groznica
Dental caries	Zubni karijes
Dental plaque (dental tartar)	Zubni kamenac
Depression	Depresija
DeQuervain syndrome	Sindrom bubnjarskog palca (Morbus DeQuervain)
Dermatitis herpetiformis (Duhring's disease)	Duhringova bolest (dermatitis herpetiformis)
Dermatomycosis	Dermatomikoza
Dermatomyositis	Dermatomiozitis
Dermoid cyst	Dermoidna cista
Development anomalies	Razvojne anomalije
Diabetes	Dijabetes
Diabetes insipidus	Dijabetes insipidus
Diabetes mellitus	Dijabetes melitus
Diabetes mellitus type 1	Dijabetes melitus tip 1
Diabetes mellitus type 2	Dijabetes melitus tip 2
Diabetic coma	Dijabetična koma
Diabetic ketoacidosis	Dijabetična ketoacidoza
Diabetic nephropathy	Dijabetična nefropatija
Diabetic neuropathy	Dijabetična neuropatija
Diabetic retinopathy	Dijabetična retinopatija
Diaphragmatic hernia	Dijafragmalna kila
Diaphyseal humeral fracture	Prijelom nadlaktice u području dijafize
Diaphyseal tightbone fracture	Prijelom dijafize bedrene kosti
Diarrhea	Proljev (dijarea)
Difficult defecation (tenesmus)	Otežano pražnjenje crijeva (otežana defekacija)
Difficult urination (dysuria)	Otežano usporeno mokrenje (dizurija)
Difficult swallowing (dysphagia)	Otežano gutanje (disfagija)
Dilated cardiomyopathy	Dilatacijska kardiomiopatija
Diphtheria	Difterija
Discarthrosis (degenerative disc disease)	Diskartroza
Discharge	Iscjedak
Diseases of the aorta	Bolesti aorte
Dislocated ankle joint	Iščašenje skočnog zgloba
Dislocated fragments	Dislokacija ulomaka
Dislocated shoulder	Iščašenje ramena
Dislocation (luxation)	Iščašenje (dislokacija, luksacija)
Dislocation of a hip	Iščašenje kuka
Disorientation	Dezorijentiranost

Disseminated intravascular coagulation	Diseminirana intravaskularna koagulacija
Distal radial fracture	Prijelom palčane kosti loco typico
Diverticulitis	Divertikulitis
Diverticulosis	Divertikuloza
Diverticulum	Divertikul
Dizziness (vertigo)	Vrtoglavica
Dog bite	Ugriz psa
Double vision (diplopia)	Dvoslike
Down syndrome	Downov sindrom (mongoloidizam)
Dracunculiasis	Drakunkulijaza
Drooling (ptyalism, sialorrhea, slobbering)	Slinjenje
Drooping of the upper eyelid (blepharoptosis)	Spušteni kapak (blefaroptoza)
Drowning	Utapanje
Drug addiction	Ovisnost o drogama
Drug allergy	Alergija na lijekove
Drug overdose	Predoziranje drogom
Dry cough	Suhi kašalj
Dry eyes (keratoconjuctivitis sicca)	Suhe oči (kseroftalmija)
Dry gangrene	Suha gangrena
Dry mouth (xerostomia)	Suha sluznica usta
Duchenne muscular dystrophy	Duchenneova mišićna distrofija
Ductus arteriosus (ductus Botalli shunt)	Ductus Botalli
Dull pain	Tupa bol
Dullness in limbs	Tupost u udovima
Duodenal atresia	Atrezija dvanaesnika
Duodenal diverticulum	Divertikul na dvanaesniku
Duodenal ulcer	Čir na dvanaesniku
Dupuytren's contracture	Dupuytrenova kontraktura
Dust allergy	Alergija na prašinu
Dwarfism (nanism)	Patuljasti rast (nanizam)
Dyschondroplasia	Dishondroplazija
Dysentery (flux)	Dizenterija
Dysgerminoma	Disgerminom
Dyshidrosis	Dishidroza
Dyslexia	Disleksija
Dyspepsia (upset stomach)	Dispepsija (nervozni želudac)
Dystonia	Distonija
Dystrophy	Distrofija
Ear bleeding	Krvarenje iz uha
Ear pain (otalgia)	Bol u uhu (otalgija)
Early symptom (prodrome)	Predsimptom bolesti prije nego se bolest razvije
Eating disorder	Poremećaj ishrane
Ebola hemorrhagic fever	Groznica Ebola
Echinococcosis (hydatid disease)	Ehinokokoza
Echolalia	Eholalija
Echopraxia (involuntary repetition ofthe observed movements of another person)	Ehopraksija (nevoljno ponavljanje tuđih pokreta)
Ectopic pregnancy (extrauterine pregnancy)	Izvanmaternična trudnoća (ektopična trudnoća)
Eczema	Ekcem
Edema	Edem
Edwards syndrome (trisomy 18)	Trisomija 18D (Edwardsov sindrom)
Eisenmenger's syndrome	Eisenmengerov sindrom
Elbow arthrosis	Artroza lakta
Elbow dislocation (luxation of the elbow)	Iščašenje lakta
Electric shock burn	Opeklina od strujnog udara
Electrical injuries (electric shock)	Ozljede električnom strujom (strujni udar)
Electromagnetic hypersensitivity	Elektromagnetska hipersenzibilnost
Elephantiasis (lymphedema)	Elefantijaza (limfedem)
Elevated body temperature	Povišena tjelesna temperatura
Embolism	Embolija
Embryonal carcinoma	Embrionalni karcinom
Emphysema	Emfizem
Empyema	Empijem
Encephalocele	Encefalokela
Encephalopathy	Encefalopatija
Enchondroma	Enhondrom
Encopresis	Enkopreza
Endocardial fibroelastosis	Fibroelastoza endokarda
Endometrial carcinoma	Karcinom endometrija
Endometrial hyperplasia	Hiperplazija endometrija
Endometrial polyp (uterine polyp)	Polip maternice
Endometriosis	Endometrioza
Endotoxic shock	Endotoksični šok
Enlarged liver (hepatomegaly)	Povećanje jetre (hepatomegalija)
Enlarged lymph nodes (lymphadenopathy)	Povećanje limfnih čvorova (limfadenopatija)
Enlarged pupils	Proširene zjenice

Enlarged tongue	Uvećani jezik	**Extensor tendinitis**	Tendinitis
(macroglossia)	(makroglosija)	**(inflammation of**	ekstenzora prstiju
Enthesopathy	Entezopatija	**the extensor**	stopala
Eosinophilia	Eozinofilija	**tendons of the toes)**	
Ependymoma	Ependimom	**External abdominal**	Kila vanjske trbušne
Epicondylar elbow	Prijelom kondila	**wall hernia**	stijenke
fracture	nadlaktične kosti	**External bleeding**	Vanjsko krvarenje
Epidemic typhus	Trbušni tifus	**Extrajoint**	Izvanzglobni
(louse-borne	(epidemjski tifus,	**rheumatism**	reumatizam
typhus)	pjegavac)	**Facial spasm**	Grč mišića lica
Epidural bleeding	Epiduralno krvarenje	**Familial**	Obiteljska
Epidural hematoma	Epiduralni hematom	**Mediterranean**	mediteranska
Epigastric pain	Bol u epigastriju	**fever**	groznica
Epilepsy	Epilepsija	**Farmer's lung**	Farmerska pluća
Epiphyseolysis	Epifizeoliza glave	**Farsightedness**	Dalekovidnost
capitis femoris	bedrene kosti	**(hyperopia)**	
Epispadias	Epispadija	**Fat embolism**	Masna embolija
Epithelial	Karcinom	**Fatigue (exhaustion,**	Iscrpljenost (umor,
carcinoma	pokrovnog epitela	**lethargy)**	fatigo)
Erysipelas (Ignis	Crveni vjetar	**Fatty liver**	Masna metarmofoza
sacer, St. Anthony's	(vrbanac, erizipel)	**metamorphosis**	jetre
fire)		**Favus**	Tinea favosa (favus)
Erysipeloid	Erizipeloid	**Feather allergy**	Alergija na perje
Erythromelalgia	Eritromelalgija	**Febrile convulsions**	Febrilne konvulzije
(acromelalgia)		**Femoral neck**	Prijelom vrata
Erythroplakia	Eritroplazija	**fracture**	bedrene kosti
(erythroplasia)		**Fetal alcohol**	Fetusni alkoholni
Erythroplasia of	Eritroplazija Queyrat	**syndrome**	sindrom
Queyrat		**Fever**	Groznica (vrućica)
Esophageal atresia	Atrezija jednjaka	**Fibrinoid necrosis**	Fibrinoidna nekroza
Esophageal stenosis	Stenoza jednjaka	**Fibroadenoma**	Fibroadenom
Esophageal varices	Proširene vene	**Fibrocystic breast**	Fibrocistična bolest
	jednjaka	**disease**	dojke
	(flebektazije)	**Fibroma**	Fibrom
Essential	Esencijalna	**Fibromyalgia**	Fibromialgija
hypertension	hipertenzija	**Fibrosarcoma**	Fibrosarkom
Estrogen deficiency	Manjak estrogena	**(fibroblastic**	
Ewing's sarcoma	Ewing sarkom	**sarcoma)**	
	(endoteliosarkom)	**Fibrosis**	Fibroza
Exanthem	Egzantem	**Fibrous dysplasia**	Fibrozna displazija
Exanthema subitum	Rozeola infantum	**Fibrous**	Fibrozni histiocitom
(roseola infantum,	(egzantema subitum,	**histiocytoma**	
sixth disease)	šesta bolest)	**Filariasis**	Filarijaza
Exasperation	Razdražljivost	**Finger clubbing**	Batićasti prsti
Excessive hunger	Neumjerena glad	**(digital clubbing)**	
(polyphagia)		**First menstrual**	Prva mjesečnica
Excessive secretion	Pojačano lučenje	**cycle (menarche)**	(menarha)
of saliva	sline	**Fish poisoning**	Trovanje ribom
(hypersalivation)	(hipersalivacija)	**Fistula**	Fistula
Excessive sweating	Prekomjerno	**Flaccid muscle**	Mlohavi mišić
(hyperhidrosis)	znojenje	**(untoned muscle)**	
	(hiperhidroza)	**Flat foot (pes**	Spušteno stopalo
Exostosis	Egzostoza	**planus)**	(pes planus)
Expectoration of	Iskašljavanje krvi	**Floating kidney**	Spušteni bubreg
blood (hemoptysis)	(hemoptiza,	**(nephroptosis, renal**	(putujući bubreg,
	hemptoja)	**ptosis)**	nefroptoza)
Explosive wound	Eksplozivna rana	**Floppy infant**	Sindrom mlohavog
Expulsion of	Vraćanje hrane iz	**syndrome**	djeteta
undigested food	želuca u usta	**Flu (influenza)**	Gripa (influenca)
from stomack to the	(regurgitacija)	**Foamy sputum**	Pjenušavi ispljuvak
mouth		**Folliculitis**	Folikulitis
(regurgitation)		**Food allergy**	Alergija na hranu

Food aversion	Gađenje prema hrani	Glioblastoma	Glioblastom
Food poisoning	Trovanje hranom	Glioma	Gliom
Foot arthrosis	Artroza stopala	Gliosis	Glioza
Foot deformity	Deformacija stopala	Glomerulonephritis	Glomerulonefritis
Forearm tendinitis	Veslačka podlaktica (tendinitis podlaktice)	Glomus tumor (glomangioma)	Glomus-tumor
Foreign body in ear	Strano tijelo u uhu	Glucose in urine (glycosuria)	Šećer u urinu (glikozurija)
Foreign body in nose	Strano tijelo u nosu	Gluten intolerance	Nepodnošenje glutena
Fournier gangrene	Fournierova gangrena	Goiter	Guša (struma)
		Gonadoblastoma	Gonadoblastom
Fracture with displacement	Prijelom kosti s pomakom	Gonorrhea	Gonoreja (kapavac, triper)
Freiberg's disease	Freibergova bolest	Goodpasture's syndrome	Goodpastureov sindrom
Frequent urination	Učestalo mokrenje		
Frequent urination at night (nocturia)	Noćno mokrenje (nokturija)	Gout (gouty arthritis)	Ulozi (giht)
Frigidity	Frigidnost	Granulocytosis	Granulocitoza
Frostbite	Ozeblina	Granulomatous inflammation	Granulomatozna upala (granulom)
Frozen shoulder (adhesive capsulitis of shoulder)	Sindrom bolnog ramena (adhezivni kapsulitis ramena, smrznuto rame)	Granulosa cell tumor	Granuloza tumor
		Green stool	Zelenkasta stolica
Fungal infection	Gljivična infekcija	Greenstick fracture	Prijelom mlade kosti
Fungal osteomyelitis	Gljivični osteomijelitis	Groin pain syndrome	Sindrom bolnih prepona
Fur allergy	Alergija na životinjsku dlaku	Guillain-Barré syndrome	Guillain-Barréov sindrom
Furuncle (boil)	Furunkul (čir na koži)	Gunshot wound	Prostrijelna rana
		Gymnastics lower back pain	Gimnastičarska bolna križa
Gaining weight	Debljanje		
Galactorrhea	Galaktoreja	Gynecomastia	Ginekomastija
Gallbladder hydrops	Hidrops žučnog mjehura	Haglund's disease	Haglundova bolest
		Hallucination	Halucinacija
Gallstone (cholelithiasis)	Žučni kamenac (holelitijaza)	Hand and finger joints dislocation	Iščašenje zglobova šake i prstiju
Gambling addiction (ludomania)	Ovisnost o kockanju (ludopatija)	Hand arthrosis	Artroza šake
		Hand fibrositis	Fibrozitis šake
Gangrene	Gangrena	Hand tremor	Drhtanje ruku
Gas gangrene	Plinska gangrena	Hand-arm vibration syndrome (vibration white finger)	Vibracijski sindrom šaka-ruka
Gas poisoning	Trovanje plinom		
Gastric carcinoma	Karcinom želuca		
Gastric ulcer	Čir na želucu		
Gastroenteritis	Gastroenteritis	Hard of hearing	Nagluhost
Generalized edema (anasarca)	Generalizirani edem (anasarka)	Hashimoto's disease	Hashimotov sindrom
Genital herpes	Genitalni herpes	Head and brain injuries	Ozljede glave i mozga
Genital wart	Genitalna bradavica (venerična bradavica)	Headache	Glavobolja
		Hearing disorder	Poremećaj sluha
German measles (rubella)	Rubeola (crljenac)	Hearing loss	Gubitak sluha
		Heart attack (myocardial infarction)	Infarkt miokarda
Giant cell arteritis (temporal arteritis)	Arteritis divovskih stanica (temporalni arteritis)		
		Heart disease (cardiopathy)	Srčana bolest (kardiopatija)
Gigantism	Divovski stas	Heart murmur	Šum na srcu
Gigantocellular tumor (osteoclastoma)	Gigantocelularni tumor (osteoklastom)	Heart valve diseases	Bolesti srčanih zalistaka
Glanders	Sakagija	Heartburn	Žgaravica
Glaucoma	Glaukom		

Heavy metal poisoning	Trovanje teškim metalima	High blood pressure (hypertension)	Visoki krvni tlak (hipertenzija)
Heberden's nodes	Heberdenovi čvorići	High blood sugar (hyperglicemia)	Povišeni šećer u krvi (hiperglikemija)
Heel spur (calcaneal spur)	Petni trn	Hip arthrosis	Artroza kuka (koksartroza)
Hemangioendotheli-oma	Hemangioendoteli-om	Hirschsprung's disease (congenital aganglionic megacolon)	Hirschsprungova bolest (kongenitalni aganglionarni megakolon)
Hemangioma	Hemangiom		
Hematoma	Hematom		
Hemivertebrae	Hemivertebra		
Hemochromatosis	Hemokromatoza	Hirsutism	Hirzutizam
Hemoglobin in urine (hemoglobinuria)	Hemoglobin u urinu (hemoglobinurija)	Histoplasmosis (Darling's disease)	Histoplazmoza
Hemolytic anemia	Hemolitična anemija	Hives (urticaria)	Koprivnjača (urtikarija)
Hemophilia	Hemofilija	Hoarseness	Promuklost
Hemophiliac arthropathy	Hemofilična artropatija	Hodgkin's disease	Hodgkinova bolest
		Hoffa's disease	Morbus Hoffa
Hemopneumotho-rax	Hemopneumotoraks	Horseshoe kidney (renal fusion)	Potkovičasti bubreg
Hemorrhagic brain infarction	Hemoragijski infarkt mozga	Hot flushes	Valovi vrućine (valunzi)
Hemorrhagic fever with renal syndrome (Korean hemorrhagic fever)	Hemoragijska groznica s renalnim sindromom (korejska hemoragijska groznica)	Human bite	Ugriz čovjeka (ljudski ugriz)
		Human papilloma virus (HPV) infection	Infekcija humanim papiloma virusom (HPV)
Hemorrhoids	Hemoroidi	Humeral neck fracture	Prijelom vrata nadlaktične kosti
Hemosiderosis	Hemosideroza	Hunchback	Grba
Hemothorax	Hemotoraks	Hunger	Glad
Hepatic echinococcosis	Ehinokokoza jetre	Huntington's chorea (Huntington's disease)	Huntingtonova koreja
Hepatic tuberculosis	Tuberkuloza jetre		
Hepatitis A	Hepatitis A	Hyaline membrane disease (infant respiratory distress syndrome)	Bolest hijaline membrane (respiratorni sindrom novorođenčeta)
Hepatitis B	Hepatitis B		
Hepatitis C	Hepatitis C		
Hepatitis D	Hepatitis D		
Hepatitis E	Hepatitis E		
Hepatocellular adenoma	Hepatocelularni adenom	Hydremia	Hidremija
		Hydrocele	Hidrokela
Hepatocellular carcinoma	Hepatocelularni karcinom	Hydrocephalus	Hidrocefalus
		Hydronephrosis	Hidronefroza
Hepatorenal syndrome	Hepatorenalni sindrom	Hydrops	Hidrops
		Hydrothorax	Hidrotoraks
Hereditary ataxia	Heredoataksija	Hygroma	Higrom
Hereditary multiple exostoses	Multiple egzostoze	Hyperactivity	Hiperaktivnost
		Hypercalcemia	Hiperkalcijemija
Hermaphroditism	Dvospolnost	Hyperinsulinism	Povišen inzulin u krvi (hiperinzulinizam)
Hernia	Kila (bruh, hernija)		
Hernia sack	Kilna vreća		
Herpangina (mouth blisters)	Herpangina	Hyperkalemia	Hiperkalijemija
		Hyperparathyroi-dism	Hiperparatireoidizam
Herpes simplex	Herpes simpleks		
Herpes zoster	Herpes zoster	Hyperpituitarism	Hiperpituitarizam
Hiatus hernia	Hijatusna kila	Hyperthermia	Hipertermija
Hiccup	Štucavica	Hyperthropic osteoarthropaty (Pierre Marie-Bamberger syndrome)	Osteoartropatija hipertrofika Pierre Marie
High arches (pes cavus)	Izdubljeno stopalo (pes excavatus)		
High blood cholesterol (hyper-cholesterolemia)	Povišeni kolesterol u krvi (hiperkolestero-lemija)		
		Hyperthyroidism	Hipertireoza

Hypertrophic cardiomyopathy	Hipertrofijska kardiomiopatija	Increased thirst senasation (polydipsia)	Pojačan osjećaj žeđi (polidipsija)
Hypertrophic pyloric stenosis	Hipertrofijska stenoza pilorusa	Indigestion	Probavne smetnje
Hypertrophy	Hipertrofija	Infarct	Infarkt
Hyperuricemia	Hiperurikemija	Infected mosquito bite	Ugriz zaraženog komarca
Hyperventilation	Hiperventilacija		
Hypervitaminosis	Hipervitaminoza	Infected tick bite	Ugriz zaraženog krpelja
Hypervolemia (increased level of fluid in the blood)	Hipervolemija (porast volumena krvi u optoku)	Infection	Infekcija
Hyphema	Hifema	Infection of the bone or bone marrow (osteomyelitis)	Infekcija kosti ili koštane srži (osteomijelitis)
Hypoalbuminemia	Hipoalbuminemija		
Hypocalcemia	Hipokalcijemija		
Hypochondria	Hipohondrija	Infectious arthritis (septic arthritis)	Infekcijski artritis (septički artritis)
Hypochromic anemia	Hipokromna anemija		
Hypoglycemia	Hipoglikemija	Infectious erythema (fifth disease)	Infektivni eritem (peta bolest)
Hypoinsulinism	Hipoinzulinizam	Infectious mononucleosis (Pfeiffer's disease, kissing disease, glandular fever)	Mononukleoza (bolest poljupca)
Hypokalemia	Hipokalijemija		
Hypoparathyroidism	Hipoparatireodizam		
Hypopituitarism	Hipopituitarizam		
Hypospadias	Hipospadija		
Hypotension and syncope	Hipotenzija i sinkope	Infertility (sterility)	Neplodnost (sterilitet)
Hypothermia	Pothlađenost (hipotermija)	Infestation with head lice (pediculosis)	Infestacija ušima (ušljivost, pedikuloza)
Hypothyroidism	Hipotireoza	Infestation with intestinal parasitic warms (helminthiasis)	Infestacija crijevnim parazitima (helmintijaza)
Hypotonia	Hipotonija		
Hypovolemic shock	Hipovolemički šok		
Hypoxia	Hipoksija		
Hysteria	Histerija	Infestation with pubic lice (phthiriasis)	Infestacija stidnim ušima (iftirijaza)
Idiopathic pulmonary fibrosis	Plućna idiopatska fibroza		
Ileus	Ileus	Inflammation	Upala
Iliotibial band friction syndrome	Sindrom trenja iliotibijalnog traktusa	Inflammation of the appendix (appendicitis)	Upala slijepog crijeva (apendicitis)
Imbecility	Slaboumnost		
Immunodeficiency	Sniženi imunitet	Inflammation of the arterial walls (arteritis)	Upala stijenke arterije (arteritis)
Impacted cerumen	Ceruminozni čep		
Impetigo	Impetigo		
Impotency	Impotencija	Inflammation of the brain (encephalitis)	Upala mozga (encefalitis)
Inability to urinate	Nemogućnost mokrenja		
Incomplete fracture	Nepotpuni prijelom kosti (napuknuće kosti)	Inflammation of the breast (mastitis)	Upala dojke (mastitis)
		Inflammation of the bronchi (bronchitis)	Upala bronhija (bronhitis)
Incontinence	Inkontinencija	Inflammation of the bronchioles (bronchiolitis)	Upala bronhiola (bronhiolitis)
Increased distance between two organs or parts of the body (hypertelorism)	Povećan razmak između dva organa ili dijela tijela (hipertelorizam)		
		Inflammation of the conjunctiva (conjunctivitis)	Upala sluznice oka (konjuktivitis)
Increased hair loss	Pojačano opadanje kose		
Increased hairiness (hypertrichosis)	Pojačana dlakavost	Inflammation of the cornea (keratitis)	Upala rožnice (keratitis)
Increased sensitivity to stimuli of the senses (hyperesthesia)	Preosjetljivost na podražaj (hiperestezija)	Inflammation of the cornea and conjunctiva (keratoconjunctivitis)	Upala rožnice i sluznice oka (keratokonjuktivitis)

Inflammation of the endocardium (endocarditis) — Upala srčane ovojnice (endokarditis)

Inflammation of the endometrium (endometritis) — Upala endometrija maternice (endometritis)

Inflammation of the enthesis (enthesitis) — Upala hvatišta mišića (entezitis)

Inflammation of the epididymis (epididymitis) — Upala pasjemenika (epididimitis)

Inflammation of the epiglottis (epiglottitis) — Upala epiglotisa (epiglotitis)

Inflammation of the fascia (fasciitis) — Upala fascije (fasciitis)

Inflammation of the gall bladder (cholecystitis) — Upala žučnog mjehura (holecistitis)

Inflammation of the glans penis (balanitis) — Upala glavića penisa (balanitis)

Inflammation of the gums (gingivitis) — Upala desni (gingivitis)

Inflammation of the heart muscle (myocarditis) — Upala srčanog mišića (miokarditis)

Inflammation of the inner ear (labyrinthitis) — Upala labirinta u unutarnjem uhu (labirintitis)

Inflammation of the joint (arthritis) — Upala zgloba (artritis)

Inflammation of the kidney (nephritis) — Upala bubrega (nefritis)

Inflammation of the larynx (laryngitis) — Upala glasnica (laringitis)

Inflammation of the liver (hepatitis) — Upala jetre (hepatitis)

Inflammation of the lung (pneumonia) — Upala pluća (pneumonija)

Inflammation of the lymph node (lymphadenitis) — Upala limfnog čvora (limfadenitis)

Inflammation of the meninges (meningitis) — Upala moždanih ovojnica (meningitis)

Inflammation of the middle layer of the eye (uveitis) — Upala srednje ovojnice oka (uveitis)

Inflammation of the mouth mucous lining (stomatitis) — Upala sluznice usta (stomatitis)

Inflammation of the muscles (myositis) — Upala mišića (miozitis)

Inflammation of the nerve (neuritis) — Upala živca (neuritis)

Inflammation of the pancreas (pancreatitis) — Upala gušterače (pankreatitis)

Inflammation of the parametrium (parametritis) — Upala parametrija (parametritis)

Inflammation of the paranasal sinuses (sinusitis) — Upala sinusa (sinusitis)

Inflammation of the pericardium (pericarditis) — Upala osrčja (perikarditis)

Inflammation of the peritoneum (peritonitis) — Upala potrbušnice (peritonitis)

Inflammation of the pleura (pleuritis) — Upala plućne ovojnice (pleuritis)

Inflammation of the prostate gland (prostatitis) — Upala prostate (prostatitis)

Inflammation of the retina (retinitis) — Upala mrežnice (retinitis)

Inflammation of the salivary gland (sialadenitis) — Upala žlijezda slinovnica (sialadenitis)

Inflammation of the skin (dermatitis) — Upala kože (dermatitis)

Inflammation of the stomach lining (gastritis) — Upala želučane sluznice (gastritis)

Inflammation of the synovial fluid sac (bursitis) — Upala sluzne vreće (burzitis)

Inflammation of the synovial membrane (synovitis) — Upala tetivne ovojnice (sinovitis)

Inflammation of the synovium and tendon (tenosynovitis) — Upala tetive s ovojnicom (tenosinovitis)

Inflammation of the tendon (tendinitis, tendonitis) — Upala tetive (tendinitis)

Inflammation of the testes (orchitis) — Upala testisa (orhitis)

Inflammation of the thymus (thymitis) — Upala prsne žlijezde (timitis)

Inflammation of the thyroid gland (thyroiditis) — Upala štitnjače (tireoiditis)

Inflammation of the tonsils (tonsillitis) — Upala krajnika (tonzilitis)

Inflammation of the urethra (urethritis) — Upala sluznice mokraćne cijevi (uretritis)

Inflammation of the urinary bladder (cystitis) — Upala mokraćnog mjehura (cistitis)

Inflammation of the vagina (vaginitis) — Upala rodnice (vaginitis)

Inflammation of the vein (phlebitis) — Upala vena (flebitis)

Inflammation of the vulva (vulvitis) — Upala stidnice (vulvitis)

Inflammation of the windpipe (tracheitis) — Upala dušnika (traheitis)

Ingrown nail (onychocryptosis, unguis incarnatus)	Urasli nokat (ungvis inkarnatus)
Inguinal hernia	Preponska kila
Insecticide poisoning	Trovanje insekticidima
Insomnia	Nesanica
Intermittent claudication	Intermitentna klaudikacija
Internal bleeding	Unutarnje krvarenje
Interstitial lung disease	Intersticijska bolest pluća
Interstitial nephritis	Intersticijska upala bubrega
Intestinal atresia	Crijevna atrezija
Intestinal tuberculosis	Tuberkuloza crijeva
Intracerebral hematoma	Intracerebralni hematom
Intracerebral hemorrhage	Intracerebralno krvarenje
Intracranial hypertension	Intrakranijalna hipertenzija
Inverted nipple	Uvućena bradavica
Involuntary swearing (coprolalia)	Nekontrolirano psovanje (koprolalija)
Ionising irradiation	Ionizirajuća ozračenost
Iridodialysis (coredialysis)	Iridodijaliza
Iritis	Iritis
Iron deficiency anemia (sideropenic anemia)	Anemija radi deficita željeza (sideropenična anemija)
Iron poisoning	Trovanje željezom
Irritable bowel syndrome (spastic colon)	Sindrom iritabilnog crijeva (spastični kolon)
Irritant contact dermatitis	Iritantni kontaktni dermatitis
Irritated knee (jumper's knee, patellar tendinopathy)	Podraženo koljeno (skakačko koljeno)
Ischemia	Ishemija
Ischemic heart disease	Ishemijska bolest srca
Ischemic limbs	Ishemični udovi
Ischemic ulceration	Ishemična ulceracija
Isosporiasis	Izosporijaza
Itching	Svrbež
Jaundice (icterus)	Žutica (ikterus)
Jellyfish sting burn	Opeklina od meduze
Joint contracture	Kontraktura zgloba
Joint distortion	Uganuće zgloba (distorzija zgloba)
Joint pain (arthralgia)	Bol u zglobu (artralgija)
Joint stiffness	Zakočenost zgloba
Juvenile osteochondrosis	Juvenilna osteohondroza
Juvenile rheumatoid arthritis	Mladenački reumatoidni artritis (juvenilni reumatoidni artritis)
Kala-azar (black fever)	Kala-azar
Kaposi's sarcoma	Kaposijev sarkom (endoteliosarkom)
Kawasaki disease	Kawasakijeva bolest (mukokutani limfoglandularni sindrom)
Keloid	Keloid
Keratosis	Keratoza
Kernicterus	Žutica moždanih jezgri
Kidney failure (renal insufficiency)	Zatajenje bubrega (insuficijencija bubrega)
Kidney stone (nephrolithiasis)	Bubrežni kamenac (nefrolitijaza)
Kidney transplatation	Transplantacija bubrega
Kienböck's disease	Kienböckova bolest
Kleptomania	Kleptomanija
Knee arthrosis	Artroza koljena (gonartroza)
Knee dislocation (luxation of the knee)	Iščašenje koljena
Knock knees (genu valgum)	Genu valgum
Knot (lump)	Kvržica
Köhler disease	Köhlerova bolest
Koplik's spots	Koplikove pjege
Kuru	Kuru (smrtni smijeh)
Kussmaul breathing	Kussmaulovo disanje
Kyphoscoliosis	Kifoskolioza
Kyphosis	Kifoza
Laceration (tear)	Razderotina
Lack of coordination of muscle movements (ataxia)	Poremećaj koordinacije mišićnih pokreta (ataksija)
Lactose intolerance	Nepodnošenje laktoze (netolerancija laktoze)
Lambliasis (giardiasis)	Lamblijaza (giardijaza)
Laryngospasm	Laringospazam
Lassa fever	Groznica Lassa
Lazy eye (amblyopia)	Slabovidnost
Lead poisoning	Trovanje olovom
Leakage of cerebrospinal fluid through the ear	Curenje likvora na uho (cerebrospinalna otoreja)

Leakage of cerebrospinal fluid through the nose	Curenje likvora na nos (cerebrospinalna rinoreja)
Learning disability	Poremećaj učenja
Leg varicose veins	Proširene vene na nogama
Legg-Calvé-Perthes disease	Legg-Calvé-Perthesova bolest
Leiomyoma	Lejomiom
Leiomyosarcoma	Lejomiosarkom
Leishmaniasis	Lišmenijaza
Leprosy	Lepra (guba)
Leptospirosis	Leptospiroza
Leukemia	Leukemija
Leukocytosis	Leukocitoza
Leukodystrophy	Leukodistrofija
Leukoplakia	Leukoplakija
Leukorrhea	Bijelo pranje
Lichen planus	Lišaj (lichen planus)
Ligament rupture (torn ligament)	Puknuće ligamenta
Ligament sprain	Istegnuće ligamenta
Limited joint mobility	Ograničena pokretljivost zgloba
Limping	Šepanje
Lipodystrophy	Lipodistrofija
Lipoma	Lipom
Liposarcoma	Liposarkom
Listeriosis	Listerioza
Lithium poisoning	Trovanje litijem
Little league elbow syndrome (LLE syndrome)	Sindrom kopljaškog lakta
Liver abscess	Apsces jetre
Liver cirrhosis	Ciroza jetre
Liver insufficiency	Zatajenje jetre
Long-lasting painful erection (priapism)	Dugotrajna bolna erekcija (prijapizam)
Lordosis	Lordoza
Loss of appetite	Gubitak apetita
Loss of half of a field of vision (hemianopsia)	Gubitak polovice vidnog polja (hemianopsija)
Loss of language ability (aphasia)	Gubitak sposobnosti govora (afazija)
Loss of olfaction (anosmia)	Gubitak osjeta mirisa
Loss of strenght (asthenia)	Gubitak mišićne snage (astenija)
Loss of the sense of taste (ageusia)	Gubitak osjeta okusa
Loss of the sense of touch	Gubitak osjeta dodoira
Low back pain (lumbago, lumbo-sacral syndrome)	Križobolja (lumbosakralni sindrom)
Low blood pressure (hypotension)	Nizak krvni tlak (hipotenzija)
Low semen volume (oligospermia)	Manjak sperme (oligospermija)
Luetic osteomyelitis	Luetični osteomijelitis
Lung abscess	Apsces pluća
Lupus erythematosus	Sistemski lupus eritematozus
Luxating patella (trick knee, floating patella)	Iščašenje čašice
Lyme disease (lyme borreliosis)	Lajmska bolest (Lajmska borelioza)
Lymphangioma	Limfangiom
Lymphangiosarco-ma	Limfangiosarkom
Lymphatic leukemia	Limfatična leukemija
Lymphedema	Limfedem (zastoj limfe)
Lymphocytic choriomeningitis	Limfocitni koriomeningitis
Lymphoma	Limfom
Macular degeneration	Degeneracija makule
Madelung's deformity	Madelungov deformitet
Malabsorption	Malapsorpcija
Malaria	Malarija
Malignant hypertension	Maligna hipertenzija
Malignant mixed tumor	Mješoviti maligni tumor
Malignant tumor (cancer)	Zloćudni tumor (maligni tumor, rak)
Mandibular dislocation	Iščašenje vilice
Mania	Manija
Marburg hemorrhagic fever	Marburška hemoragijska groznica
Marfan syndrome	Marfanov sindrom
Mastopathy	Mastopatija
McCune-Albright syndrome	Albrightov sindrom
Measles	Ospice (morbili)
Mechanic icterus (bile duct obstruction)	Mehanički ikterus
Mechanical injuries	Mehaničke ozljede
Medication overdose	Predoziranje lijekom
Medullary carcinoma	Medularni karcinom
Medulloblastoma	Meduloblastom
Megacolon	Megakolon
Megaloblastic anemia	Megaloblastična anemija (anemija radi deficita vitamina)
Melanoma	Melanom
Melasma (chloasma faciei)	Kloazma (melazma)
Melioidosis (Whitmore disease)	Melioidoza
Memory loss	Gubitak pamćenja
Meniere's disease	Menierova bolest

Meningioma	Meningeom	Muscle strain	Istegnuće mišića
Meningocele	Meningokela	(muscle pull)	(distenzija mišića)
Meningoencephalo-cele	Meningoencefaloke-la	Muscle twitch (fasciculation)	Trzanje mišića
Meningomyelocele	Meningomijelokela	Muscular	Kontraktura mišića
Meniscal disease	Meniskopatija	contracture	
Meniscus rupture (meniscus tear)	Razdor meniskusa	Muscular cramp (spasm)	Mišićni grč (spazam)
Menopause	Menopauza (klimakterij)	Muscular dystrophy	Mišićna distrofija
		Muscular fibrositis	Fibrozitis mišića
Menstrual disorder	Menstrualne smetnje	Muscular hypotonia	Mišićna hipotonija
Mental retardation	Mentalna retardacija	Mushroom	Trovanje gljivama
Mercury poisoning	Trovanje živom	poisoning	
Mesothelioma	Mezoteliom	Myasthenia gravis	Miastenija gravis
Metabolic acidosis	Metabolička acidoza	Mycetoma	Micetoma
Metal fume fever	Metalna groznica	Mycosis	Mikoza
Metastasis	Metastaza	Myelodysplastic	Mijelodisplastični
Metatarsalgia	Metatarzalgija	syndrome	sindrom
(Morton's neuroma)	(Mortonova metatarzalgija)	Myeloid leukemia	Mijeloična leukemija
		Myoblastoma	Mioblastom
Meteoropathy	Meteoropatija	Myoclonic twitches	Miokloničko trzanje
Methanol poisoning	Trovanje metanolom	(myoclonus)	(mioklonus)
Migraine	Migrena	Myogelosis	Miogeloza
Milia (milk spots)	Milije (dječje akne)	Myoma	Miom
Miliaria rubra (sweat rash)	Milijarija rubra	Myosarcoma	Miosarkom
		Myositis ossificans	Osificirajući miozitis
Mitral stenosis	Stenoza mitralnog ušća	Myositis ossificans progressiva	Progresivno okoštavanje mišića
Mixed tumor	Mješoviti tumor	Myxedema	Miksedem
Molluscum	Molusk	Myxoma	Miksom
contagiosum		Myxosarcoma	Miksosarkom
Monocytic leukemia	Monocitična leukemija	Nail biting (onychophagia)	Griženje noktiju (onikofagija)
Mood swing	Promjene raspoloženja	Narcolepsy	Narkolepsija
		Nasal congestion	Začepljeni nos
Morquio's syndrome (mucopolysacchari-dosis IV)	Sindrom Morquio (mukopolisaharidoza tip IV)	(stuffy nose)	
		Nasal polyp	Polip u nosu (nosni polip)
		Nasal secretion (mucus)	Sekrecija iz nosa
Motor neurone disease	Bolest motornog neurona	Nasal septum deviation	Devijacija nosnog septuma
Movement ability	Sposobnost kretanja	Natural death	Prirodna smrt
Movement disorder	Poremećaj kretanja	Nausea	Mučnina
Movement inability	Nemogućnost kretanja	Neck myalgia	Mijalgični sindrom vrata
MRSA	MRSA	Neck varicose veins	Proširene vratne vene
Mucocele	Mukocela		
Mucopolysacchari-dosis	Mukopolisaharidoza	Necrosis	Nekroza
Mucus in stool	Sluzava stolica	Necrotizing fasciitis	Nekrotizirajući fasciitis
Multiple sclerosis	Multipla skleroza		
Multiple system atrophy	Multipla sistemska atrofija	Neonatal jaundice	Novorođenačka žutica
Mumps (epidemic parotitis)	Zaušnjaci (mumps, parotitis)	Nephrosis	Nefroza
		Nephrotic syndrome	Nefrotski sindrom
Murine typhus (endemic typhus)	Štakorski pjegavac	Nerve compression (pinched nerve)	Kompresija živca (uklješten živac)
Muscle pain (myalgia)	Bol u mišiću (mijalgija)	Nerve lesion	Oštećenje živca (lezija živca)
Muscle rupture	Rastrgnuće mišića (ruptura mišića)	Neuralgia	Neuralgija
		Neurasthenia	Neurastenija

Neurinoma	Neurinom	Osteogenesis	Osteogeneza
Neuroblastoma	Neuroblastom	imperfecta (brittle	imperfekta (staklaste
Neuroborreliosis	Neuroborelioza	bone disease)	kosti)
Neurofibromatosis	Von	Osteoma	Osteom
type 1 (Von	Recklinghausenova	Osteomalacia	Osteomalacija
Recklinghausen's	bolest	Osteopetrosis	Osteopetroza
disease)		(marble bone	(zadebljane kosti,
Neurogenic shock	Neurogeni šok	disease)	bolest mramornih
Neuroma	Neurom		kostiju)
Neuropathy	Neuropatija	Osteoporosis	Osteoporoza
Neurosis	Neuroza	Osteosarcoma	Osteosa
Night blindness	Noćno sljepilo	Osteosclerosis	Osteoskleroza
(nyctalopia)		Ovarian cyst	Cista na jajniku
Night sweats	Noćno znojenje	Ovulation pain	Bolna ovulacija
Nocturnal leg	Noćni grčevi u	(mittelschmerz)	(mittelschmerz)
cramps	nogama	Paget's disease	Pagetova bolest
Nodular goiter	Čvorasta guša	Pain	Bol
	(nodularna struma)	Pain syndrome	Bolni sindrom
Non-Hodgkin's	Non-Hodgkinov	Painful	Bolna menstruacija
lymphoma	limfom	menstruation	(dismenoreja)
Non-ionising	Neionizirajuća	(dysmenorrhea)	
irradiation	ozračenost	Painful sexual	Bol pri snošaju
Nonpassage of urine	Prestanak lučenja	intercourse	
	urina	(dyspareunia)	
Nose bleeding	Krvarenje iz nosa	Painful swallowing	Bolno gutanje
(epistaxis)	(epistaksa)	(odynophagia)	(odinofagija)
Nuchal rigidity	Kočenje šije	Painful urination	Bol pri mokrenju
(stiff neck)	(ukočeni vrat)	(strangury)	(strangurija)
Numbness in limbs	Utrnulost udova	Paleness (pallor)	Bljedilo
Nummular	Numularni	Palpitation	Lupanje srca
dermatitis	dermatitis		(palpitacije)
Nystagmus	Nistagmus	Pancreatic cyst	Cista na gušterači
Obesity	Debljina (gojaznost)	Pancreatic	Lipomatoza
Oblique fracture	Kosi prijelom kosti	lipomatosis	gušterače (masna
Obstructive lesion	Opstruktivna lezija		infiltracija gusterače)
of the small	tankog crijeva	Panic attack	Napadaj panike
intestine		Panner's disease	Pannerova bolest
Obstructive shock	Opstruktivni šok	Papillary carcinoma	Papilarni karcinom
Occipital neuralgia	Okcipitalna	Papilloma	Papilom
(Arnold's neuralgia)	neuralgija	Pappataci fever	Papataći-groznica
Occupational	Profesionalno	(phlebotomus fever,	
disease	oboljenje	sandfly fever)	
Oligodendroglioma	Oligodendrogliom	Paracetamol	Trovanje
Oligomenorrhea	Oligomenoreja	poisoning	paracetamolom
Onchocerciasis	Onkocerkijaza	Paracoccidioidomy-	Parakokcidioidomi-
(river blindness)	(riječno sljepilo)	cosis (Brazilian	koza (brazilska
Open fracture	Otvoreni prijelom	blastomycosis)	blastomikoza)
(compound	kosti	Paragonimiasis	Paragonimijaza
fracture)		Paralysis	Paraliza (oduzetost,
Optic nerve edema	Otok očnog živca		kljenut)
	(zastojna papila)	Paralysis of all	Oduzetost gornjih i
Orbital cellulitis	Celulitis orbite	limbs and torso	donjih ekstremiteta i
Oroya fever	Oroya groznica	(quadriplegia,	torza (kvadriplegija,
(Carrion's disease)	(Carrionova bolest)	tetraplegia)	tetraplegija)
Osgood-Schlatter	Osgood-Schlatterova	Paralysis of lower	Oduzetost donjih
disease (rugby	bolest	extremities	ekstremiteta
knee)		(paraplegia)	(paraplegija)
Osteitis fibrosa	Fibrozna cistična	Paralysis of one half	Oduzetost jedne
cystica	upala kosti	of a body	polovine tijela
Osteochondroma	Osteohondrom	(hemiplegia)	(hemiplegija)

Paralysis of symmetrical parts of the body (diplegia)	Oduzetost simetričnih dijelova tijela (diplegija)	Petechia	Petehije
		Peyronie's disease (induratio penis plastica)	Plastična induracija penisa
Paranoia	Paranoja	Phantom pain	Fantomska bol
Parasitic disease (parasitosis)	Parazitarna bolest (parazitoza)	Phenylketonuria	Fenilketonurija
Paratyphoid fever	Trbušni paratifus	Pheochromocytoma	Feokromocitom (tumor srži nadbubrežne žlijezde)
Paresis	Pareza		
Parkinson's disease	Parkinsonova bolest		
Paronychia	Paronihija	Phimosis	Fimoza
Partial dislocation (subluxation)	Djelomična dislokacija (subluksacija)	Phlebothrombosis	Flebotromboza
		Phlegmon	Flegmona
		Phobia	Fobija
Passage of large volumes of urine (polyuria)	Učestalo mokrenje velikih količina mokraće (poliurija)	Photophobia (fear of light)	Fotofobija (strah od svjetla)
		Pig flu (swine influenza, influenzavirus A subtype H1N1)	Svinjska gripa
Passing gas (flatulence, farting)	Puštanje vjetra (flatulencija, plinovi)		
Patau syndrome (trisomy 13)	Trisomija 13D (Patauov sindrom)		
Patent ductus arteriosus (persistent ductus arteriosus)	Otvoreni ductus arteriosus (Ductus arteriosus persistens)	Pigeon chest (pectus carinatum)	Kokošja prsa
		Pilonidal cyst	Pilonidalna cista
		Pinta	Pinta
		Plague (pest)	Kuga
Pectus excavatum	Udubljena prsa (ljevkasta prsa)	Plantar fasciitis	Plantarni fasciitis
		Plasmacytoma (multiple myeloma)	Plazmocitom (multipli mijelom)
Pellegrini-Stieda disease	Bolest Pellegrini-Stieda		
		Pleural carcinosis	Karcinoza pleure
Pelvic inflammatory disease	Upalna bolest zdjelice	Pneumoconiosis	Pneumokonioza
		Pneumocystis pneumonia (pneumocystosis)	Pneumocistična upala pluća
Pemphigus	Pemfigus		
Perforated eardrum (tympanorrhexis)	Puknuće bubnjića (perforacija bubnjića, timpanoreksija)		
		Pneumothorax	Pneumotoraks
		Poisoning (toxication)	Trovanje
Perforated ulcer	Puknuće čira (perforacija ulkusa)	Poliomyelitis(polio, infantile paralysis)	Dječja paraliza (polio, poliomijelitis)
Perianal abscess	Perianalni apsces	Pollen allergy	Alergija na pelud
Pericardial carcinosis	Karcinoza perikarda	Polycystic kidney disease	Policistični bubreg
Pericardial effusion (hydropericard)	Hidroperikard	Polycythemia	Policitemija
		Polydactyly	Polidaktilija
Pericardial tamponade (cardiac tamponade)	Tamponada perikarda	Polymyalgia rheumatica	Reumatska polimialgija
		Polymyositis	Polimiozitis
		Polyp	Polip
Perinephric abscess	Paranefritički apsces	Popliteus syndrome	Sindrom m. popliteusa
Periodic breathing (Cheyne-Stokes respiration)	Periodično disanje (Cheyne-Stokesovo disanje)		
		Porphyria	Porfirija
		Portal hypertension	Portalna hipertenzija
Periodontitis	Parodontoza	Post-necrotic cirrhosis	Postnekrotična ciroza
Peripheral nerve lesion	Oštećenje perifernog živca	Post-thrombotic syndrome	Posttrombotički sindrom
Peritoneal carcinosis	Karcinoza peritoneuma	Post-traumatic headache	Posttraumatska glavobolja
Pernicious anemia	Perniciozna anemija		
Personality changes	Promjene osobnosti	Posterior ankle impingement syndrome	Sindrom sraza stražnjeg nožnog zgloba
Personality disorder	Poremećaj osobnosti		
Pes calcaneus	Petno stopalo		
Pes valgus	Izvrnuto stopalo (pes valgus)		

Posttraumatic stress disorder	Posttraumatski stresni poremećaj (PTSP)	Pulmonary infarction	Infarkt pluća
Postural back pain	Posturalna križobolja	Pulmonary tuberculosis	Tuberkuloza pluća
Postural edema	Posturalni edem (statički edem)	Pulmonary valve stenosis	Stenoza plućnog ušća (pulmonalna stenoza)
Precocious puberty (premature puberty)	Preuranjeni pubertet	Pulsing pain	Pulsirajuća bol
Preiser disease	Morbus Preiser	Purpura	Purpura
Premature ejaculation	Prijevremena ejakulacija	Pus	Gnoj
		Pus in sputum	Gnojni ispljuvak
Premature sexual development of the opposite sex	Prerano spolno fizičko sazrijevanje suprotnog spola	Pus in urine (pyuria)	Gnoj u urinu (piurija)
		Pustule	Gnojni mjehurić
Premature sexual development of the same sex	Prerano splono fizičko sazrijevanje istog spola	Pyelonephritis (kidney infection)	Pijelonefritis (infekcija bubrega)
		Pyloric stenosis	Stenoza pilorusa (pilorostenoza)
Premenstrual syndrome (PMS)	Predmenstruacijski sindrom (PMS)	Pylorospasm	Pilorospazam
		Pyonephrosis	Pionefroza
Primary amoebic meningoencephali-tis	Primarni amebni meningoencefalitis	Pyromania	Piromanija
		Q fever	Q-groznica
		Quinsy (peritonsillar abscess)	Gnojna upala krajnika
Prinzmetal's angina	Prinzmetalova angina		
Proctitis	Proktitis	Rabies	Bjesnoća (rabies)
Productive cough	Produktivni kašalj	Radial head fracture (radial capitulum fracture)	Prijelom glavice palčane kosti
Progressive muscular dystrophy	Progresivna mišićna distrofija		
Prostate cancer	Rak prostate	Radiation poisoning	Trovanje zračenjem
Prostate carcinoma	Karcinom prostate	Radioactive irradiation	Radioaktivna ozračenost
Proteinuria (presence of proteins in urine)	Bjelančevine u urinu (proteinurija)	Radioulnar synostosis	Radioulnarna sinostoza
Pseudoepithelioma-tous hyperplasia	Pseudoepieliemato-zna hiperplazija	Radius fracture	Prijelom palčane kosti
Psittacosis (parrot fever)	Psitakoza	Rapid breathing (tachypnea)	Ubrzano disanje (tahipnea)
Psoriasis	Psorijaza	Rash (eruption, eczema)	Osip
Psoriatic arthritis	Psorijatični artritis		
Psychic changes	Psihičke promjene	Rat bite	Ugriz štakora
Psychoneurosis	Psihoneuroza	Rat-bite fever	Groznica štakorskog ugriza
Psychopathy	Psihopatija		
Psychosis	Psihoza	Raynaud's disease	Raynaudova bolest
Pulmonary alveolar proteinosis	Alveolarna proteinoza pluća	Reactive arthritis (Reiter's syndrome)	Reiterov sindrom
Pulmonary atelectasis	Atelektaza pluća	Rectal prolapse	Prolaps rektuma
Pulmonary congestion	Plućna kongestija	Red colored stool	Crvena stolica
		Red urine	Crveni urin
Pulmonary echinococcosis	Ehinokokoza pluća	Redness of the skin (erythema)	Crvenilo kože (eritem)
Pulmonary edema	Plućni edem	Refracturing (repeated fracture)	Opetovani prijelom kosti
Pulmonary embolism	Plućna embolija		
Pulmonary heart disease	Plućno srce	Relapsing fever	Povratna groznica
		Renal agenesis	Agenezija bubrega
Pulmonary hypertension	Plućna hipertenzija	Renal cell carcinoma (hypernephroma)	Hipernefrom
Pulmonary hypoplasia	Hipoplazija plućnog režnja	Renal colic	Bubrežna kolika (renalna kolika)
		Renal cyst	Cista na bubregu

Renal rickets	Bubrežni rahitis	Runny nose (rinorrhea)	Curenje iz nosa (rinoreja)
Renal tuberculosis	Tuberkuloza bubrega	Rupture	Prsnuće (puknuće, razdor, ruptura)
Renal tubular acidosis	Renalna tubularna acidoza		
Renovacsular hypertension	Renovaskularna hipertenzija	Rupture of urinary bladder	Rascjep mokraćnog mjehura
Repetitive strain injury (cumulative trauma disorder)	Sindrom prenaprezanja	Ruptured spleen	Ruptura slezene
		Salicylate poisoning	Trovanje salicilatima
		Salmonellosis	Salmoneloza
Respiratory alkalosis	Respiratorna alkaloza	Sarcoidosis (sarcoid, Besnier-Boeck disease)	Sarkoidoza
Respiratory distress syndrome	Respiratorni distres sindrom	Sarcoma	Sarkom
Restrictive cardiomyopathy	Restriktivna kardiomiopatija	Sarcomatoid mesothelioma	Mezoteliosarkom
Reticuloendothelial sarcoma	Retikuloendotelijalni sarkom	Sarcopenia	Sarkopenija
		Scabies (the itch)	Svrab (skabijes)
Retinal ablation (retinal detachment)	Odvajanje mrežnice (ablacija retine)	Scar	Ožiljak
		Scarlet fever	Šarlah (skarlatina)
Retinal artery occlusion	Blokada mrežnične arterije	Schistosomiasis (snail fever)	Šistosomijaza
Retinal degeneration	Degeneracija mrežnice	Schizophrenia	Šizofrenija
		Sciatica	Išijas
Retinitis pigmentosa (retinal pigment epithelium dystrophy)	Pigmentna distrofija mrežnice	Scleroderma	Sklerodermija
		Sclerosing adenosis	Sklerozirajuća adenoza
		Scoliosis	Skolioza
		Scorpion sting	Ugriz škorpiona
Retinopathy of prematurity (retrolental fibroplasia)	Retrolentalna fibroplazija	Scotoma	Skotom
		Scratch	Ogrebotina
		Scrub typhus (Japanese river fever, Tsutsugamushi fever)	Japanska riječna groznica (Tsutsugamushi groznica)
Retroperitoneal fibrosis (Ormond's disease)	Retroperitonealna fibroza (Ormondova bolest)		
Retroverted uterus	Retrovertirani uterus	Scurvy	Skorbut
Reye's syndrome	Reyeov sindrom	Seasickness	Morska bolest
Rh incompatibility (hemolytic disease of the newborn)	Rh-inkompatibilnost (hemolitička bolest novorođenčeta)	Sebaceous cyst (wen)	Lojna cista
		Seborrhea	Seboreja
		Seborrheic keratosis	Seboreična keratoza
Rhabdomyoma	Rabdomiom	Secondary hypertension (inessential hypertension)	Sekundarna hipertenzija
Rhabdomyosarco-ma	Rabdomiosarkom		
Rheumatic fever	Reumatska groznica		
		Self-harm	Samoozljeđivanje
Rheumatic heart disease	Reumatska bolest srca	Semicoma	Semikoma
		Sensation of fear	Osjećaj straha
Rheumatoid arthritis	Reumatoidni artritis	Sensitivity to pain (algesia)	Osjetljivost na bol (algezija)
Rhinitis	Rinitis		
Rickets (rachitis)	Rahitis	Separated shoulder (acromioclavicular dislocation)	Iščašenje akromio-klavikularnog zgloba
Rickettsiosis	Rikecioza		
Riedel's thyroiditis	Riedelov tireoiditis		
Rift Valley fever	Rift Valley groznica		
Ringing in ears (tinnitus)	Zujanje u ušima (tinitus)	Sepsis	Sepsa
		Septic shock	Septički šok
Rosacea	Rozacea	Septicemia	Septikemija
Rotator cuff rupture (rotator cuff tear)	Razdor rotatorne manžete ramenog zgloba	Sever's disease	Severova bolest
		Severe acute respiratory syndrome (SARS)	Sindrom akutne respiratorne insuficijencije (SARS)
Rotten tooth	Pokvareni zub		

Sexual addiction	Ovisnost o seksu	Smallpox	Velike boginje (crne boginje, variola vera)
Sexual differentiation disorder	Poremećaj spolne diferencijacije	Snake bite	Ugriz zmije
Sexually transmitted disease	Spolno prenosiva bolest	Sneezing	Kihanje
		Sniffing (sniffle)	Šmrcanje
Shallow breathing	Površinsko plitko disanje	Soft fibroma (fibroma molle, acrochordon)	Kožni privjesak (mekani fibrom)
Sharp pain	Oštra bol		
Shedding of the skin (desquamation)	Ljuštenje kože (deskvamacija)	Somnolence	Pospanost (somnolencija)
Shellfish poisoning	Trovanje školjkašima	Sopor	Sopor
		Sore throat (inflammation of the throat, pharyngitis)	Upala grla (grlobolja, faringitis)
Shigellosis (bacillary dysentery)	Šigeloza		
Shin splints	Trkačka potkoljenica	Spanish flu	Španjolska gripa
Shivering	Zimica (tresavica)	Spasm (cramp)	Grč (spazam)
Shock	Šok	Spastic arching position (opisthotonus)	Izvijanje misića vrata i leđa u luk (opistotonus)
Shortness of breath (dyspnea)	Zaduha (nedostatak daha, dispneja)		
Shortsightedness (myopia)	Kratkovidnost	Speech difficulty (dysphasia)	Otežan govor (disfazija)
Shoulder arthrosis	Artroza ramena	Spermatocele	Spermatokela (cista epididimisa
Shoulder impingement syndrome (subacromial impingement syndrome)	Sindrom sraza ramena (subakromijalni sindrom sraza)	Spider angioma (spider nevus)	Paukoliki angiom (spider nevus)
		Spider bite	Ugriz pauka
		Spina bifida	Spina bifida
		Spinal deformity	Deformacija kralježnice
Shuffling gait	Teturav nesiguran hod	Spinal disc herniation	Hernija intervertrebralnog diska
Sickle-cell disease (sickle-cell anemia)	Anemija srpastih stanica		
		Spinal shock	Spinalni šok
Siderosis	Sideroza	Spiral fracture	Spiralni prijelom kosti
Sight disorder	Poremećaj vida		
Silicosis	Silikoza	Splenomegaly	Splenomegalija
Silo-filler's disease	Silosna pluća	Split foot (lobster claw foot, ectrodactyly)	Lobster Claw stopalo
Simple bone fracture	Jednostavni prijelom kosti		
Sinus headache	Sinusna glavobolja	Spondylitis	Spondilitis
Sister Mary Joseph nodule	Čvor sestre Mary Joseph (umbilikalna metastaza)	Spondylolisthesis	Spondilolisteza
		Spondylosis	Spondiloza
		Spontaneous fractures	Spontane frakture
Sjögren's syndrome	Sjögrenov sindrom	Sporotrichosis	Sporotrihoza
Skin color changes	Promjene boje kože	Sports injury	Sportska ozljeda
Sleep apnea	Noćna desaturacija	Sprengel's deformity	Sprengelova bolest (scapula alta)
Sleeping disorder	Poremećaj spavanja		
Sleepwalking (somnambulism)	Mjesečarenje (somnambulizam)	Squamous cell carcinoma (planocellular carcinoma)	Planocelularni karcinom
Slow basal metabolism	Usporen bazalni metabolizam		
Slow breathing rate (bradypnea)	Usporeno disanje (bradipneja)		
		Stab wound	Ubodna rana
Slow psychophysiological responses	Psihofizička usporenost	Staphylococcal food poisoning	Stafilokokno trovanje hranom
		Starvation	Izgladnjelost
Slow pulse rate (bradycardia)	Usporen puls (bradikardija)	Stenosis of pulmonary artery	Stenoza plućne arterije
Small intestine diverticulum	Divertikul tankog crijeva	Stiffness	Ukočenost
Small pupils	Sužene zjenice		

Stomach cancer (gastric cancer)	Rak želuca	Tendon rupture (torn tendon)	Puknuće tetive
Stomach growling (borborygmus)	Kruljenje u želucu	Tendon strain	Istegnuće tetive (distenzija tetive)
Strabismus	Razrokost (strabizam)	Tennis elbow	Teniski lakat
		Tension headache	Tenzijska glavobolja
Strain (sprain, pull)	Istegnuće	Teratocarcinoma	Teratokarcinom
Strangulation	Davljenje	Teratoma	Teratom
Streptococcal pharyngitis	Streptokokna angina	Testicular dysgenesis	Testikularna disgeneza
Stress fracture	Prijelom zamora	Testicular torsion	Torzija testisa
Stress urinary incontinence	Stres-inkontinencija urina	Tetanus	Tetanus (zli grč)
Stroke (cerebrovascular accident)	Moždani udar	Tetany	Tetanija
		Tetralogy of Fallot	Fallotova tetralogija
		Thalassemia	Talasemija
		Thallium poisoning	Trovanje talijem
Stupor	Stupor	Thermal injuries	Termičke ozljede
Stye (chalazion)	Ječmenac	Thermal wound	Termička rana
Subarachnoid hemorrhage	Subarahnoidalno krvarenje	Thermonuclear injuries	Termonuklearne ozljede
Subcutaneous emphysema	Potkožni emfizem	Thirst	Žed
Subdural hematoma	Subduralni hematom	Thoracic aortic aneurysm	Aneurizma torakalne aorte
Subdural hemorrhage	Subduralno krvarenje	Thoracic outlet syndrome	Torakalni sindrom
Sudden infant death syndrome (crib death, cot death)	Sindrom iznenadne smrti dojenčeta	Thrombocytopenia	Trombocitopenija
		Thromboembolism	Tromboembolija
		Thrombophlebitis	Tromboflebitis
		Thrombosis	Tromboza
Sudeck's atrophy	Sudeckova distrofija	Thrombotic thrombocytopenic purpura	Trombotska trombocitopenična purpura
Sunstroke (heat stroke)	Sunčanica		
Supracondylar femoral fracture	Suprakondilarni prijelom bedrene kosti	Thrush (oral candidiasis)	Sor (oralna kandidijaza)
		Thumb joint arthritis	Rizartroza
Supracondylar humerus fracture	Suprakondilarni prijelom nadlaktice	Thyroglossal duct cyst	Cista na tireoglosnom vodu
Supramaleolar fracture of tibia and fibula	Supramaleolarni prijelom potkoljenice	Thyroid cyst	Cista na štitnjači
		Thyrotoxicosis	Tireotoksikoza (tireotoksična oluja)
Surgical shock (postoperative shock)	Kirurški šok	Tibia stress fracture	Prijelom zamora goljenične kosti
Suspension of external breathing (apnea)	Zastoj disanja (apnea)	Tibialis posterior syndrome	Sindrom stražnjeg tibijalnog mišića
		Tibialis posterior tendinitis	Tendinitis stražnjeg tibijalnog mišića
Sweating	Znojenje	Tic	Tik
Swelling	Oteklina		
Swimmer's knee	Plivačko koljeno	Tick-borne menin-goencephalitis	Krpeljni meningoencefalitis
Syncope	Sinkopa	Tight hamstrings syndrome	Sindrom stražnje lože natkoljenice (sindrom hamstringsa)
Syndactyly	Sindaktilija		
Synovial sarcoma	Sinovijalni sarkom		
Synovioma	Sinoviom		
Syphilis	Sifilis (lues)		
Syringomyelia	Siringomijelija	'Tight shoes' sensation	Osjećaj "tijesnih cipela"
Tachycardia	Tahikardija		
Tarsal tunnel syndrome	Sindrom tarzalnog kanala	Tinea capitis (scalp ringworm)	Gljivična infekcija vlasišta (tinea capitis)
Tendinosis (chronic tendon injury)	Tendinoza (kronična ozljeda tetive)		
Tendinous fibrositis	Fibrozitis tetive	Tinea corporis	Tinea corporis

Tinea versicolor (pityriasis versicolor, haole rot)	Pitirijaza (svjetlije mrlje na osunčanoj koži, Tinea versicolor)
Tingling	Trnjenje
Tonic-clonic seizure	Toničko-klonički napadaj
Toothache	Zubobolja
Tourette's syndrome	Touretteov sindrom
Toxocariasis	Toksokarijaza
Toxoplasmosis	Toksoplazmoza
Trachoma	Trahom
Transitional cell carcinoma	Tranzicionalni karcinom
Transposition of aorta	Transpozicija aorte
Transposition of pulmonary artery	Transpozicija plućne arterije
Transposition of the great vessels	Transpozicija velikih žila
Transverse colon	Poprečno debelo crijevo
Transverse fracture	Poprečni prijelom kosti
Traumatic shock	Traumatski šok
Traveller's thrombosis (economy class syndrome)	Sindrom ekonomske klase
Tremor	Drhtanje (tremor)
Trichinosis (trichinellosis)	Trihinoza (trihineloza)
Trichomonas vaginalis	Trihomonazni vaginitis
Trichomoniasis	Trihomonijaza
Trifascicular block	Trifascikularni blok
Trigeminal neuralgia	Neuralgija trigeminusa
Trypanosomiasis	Tripanosomijaza
Tuberculosis (TBC)	Tuberkuloza (sušica, TBC)
Tuberculous arthritis	Tuberkulozni artritis
Tuberculous lymphadenitis	Tuberkuloza limfnih čvorova
Tuberculous spondylitis (Pott disease)	Tuberkulozni spondilitis (Pottova bolest)
Tubular adenoma	Tubularni adenom
Tularemia (rabbit fever)	Tularemija (zečja groznica)
Tumor (tumour)	Tumor
Tungiasis (nigua, pique)	Tungijaza
Turner syndrome	Turnerov sindrom
Twinging pain	Probadajuća bol
Typhoid fever (typhoid)	Tifusna groznica (tifus)
Ulcer	Čir (ulkus)
Ulcerative colitis	Ulcerozni kolitis
Umbilical hernia	Pupčana kila (umbilikalna hernija)
Unclear urine (foggy urine)	Mutni urin
Unconsciousness	Nesvjestica
Uncontrolled eye movement (opsoclonus)	Nekontrolirani pokreti očiju (opsoklonus)
Underfedness (malnutrition)	Neuhranjenost
Undescended testicle	Nespušteni testis
Unequal size of pupils (anisocoria)	Nejednaka veličina zjenica (anizokorija)
Upper and/or lower jaw fracture (broken upper/lower jaw)	Prijelom gornje i/ili donje čeljusti
Upper respiratory tract infection	Infekcija gornjih dišnih puteva
Uremia (autointoxication due to kidney failure)	Uremija (autointoksikacija radi nelučenja urina)
Ureteral stone (ureterolithiasis)	Ureteralni kamenac (ureterolitijaza)
Urge to vomit	Podražaj na povraćanje
Urinary burning	Pećenje za vrijeme mokrenja
Urinary incontinence	Urinarna inkotinencija
Urinary retention (ischuria)	Zastoj urina (urinarna retencija)
Urination disorder	Poremećaj mokrenja
Urogenital neoplasm	Urogenitalni tumor
Urogenital tuberculosis	Urogenitalna tuberkuloza
Uterine bleeding (metrorrhagia)	Krvarenje iz maternice (metroragija)
Uterine prolapse (fallen womb)	Prolaps maternice (spuštena maternica)
Vaginal discharge	Vaginalni iscjedak
Vaginal spasm (vaginismus)	Grč rodnice (vaginizam)
Van Neck disease	Morbus Van Neck
Varicocele	Varikokela
Varicose veins	Proširene vene
Vasomotor rhinitis	Vazomotorni rinitis
Venous bleeding	Vensko krvarenje
Venous thrombosis	Venska tromboza
Venous ulcer (varicose ulcer)	Varikozni ulcer (venski ulcer)
Ventricular fibrillation	Ventrikularna fibrilacija
Ventricular hypertrophy	Ventrikularna hipertrofija
Ventricular septal defect	Ventrikularni septalni defekt
Vibration disease	Vibracijska bolest

Violent death	Nasilna smrt
Viral conjuctivitis	Virusni konjuktivitis
Viral hemorrhagic fever	Virusna hemoragijska groznica
Viral hepatitis	Virusni hepatitis
Viral infection	Virusna infekcija
Viral pneumonia	Virusna upala pluća
Vitamin A deficiency	Manjak vitamina A
Vitamin B1 deficiency	Manjak vitamina B1
Vitamin B2 deficiency	Manjak vitamina B2
Vitamin B3 deficiency	Manjak vitamina B3
Vitamin B12 deficiency	Manjak vitamina B12
Vitamin C deficiency	Manjak vitamina C
Vitamin D deficiency	Manjak vitamina D
Vitamin deficiency	Manjak vitamina
Vitamin K deficiency	Manjak vitamina K
Vitiligo	Vitiligo
Vocal chords polyp	Polip na glasnicama
Voice changes	Promjene glasa
Volkmann's ischemic contracture	Volkmannova ishemična kontraktura
Vomiting	Povraćanje
Vomiting of blood (hematemesis)	Povraćanje krvi (hematemeza)
Vomiting without nausea (cerebral vomiting)	Povraćanje bez mučnine (povraćanje u luku, cerebralno povraćanje)
Warfare gases poisoning	Trovanje bojnim otrovima
Warm sweaty palms	Topli i vlažni dlanovi
Wart	Bradavica (virusna bradavica)
Watery eyes	Suzenje očiju
Watery stool	Vodenasta stolica
Weakness	Slabost
Weight loss (weight reduction)	Mršavljenje
West Nile fever	Groznica zapadnog Nila
Wet gangrene	Vlažna gangrena
Whipple's disease	Whippleova bolest
Whitlow (felon)	Panaricij
Whooping cough (pertussis)	Hripavac (pasji kašalj, pertussis)
Wilm's tumor (nephroblastoma)	Wilmsov tumor (nefroblastom)
Withdrawal	Apstinencijska kriza
Wound (injury, lesion)	Rana
Wrinkle	Bora

Wrist arthrosis	Artroza ručnog zgloba
Wry neck (torticollis)	Krivi vrat (tortikolis)
Xanthelasma	Ksantelazma
Xanthoma	Ksantom
Yawn	Zijevanje
Yaws (pian)	Frambezija
Yellow fever	Žuta groznica
Yellow stool	Žuta stolica
Yolk sac tumor (endodermal sinus tumor)	Tumor žumanjčane vreće (endodermalni sinus tumor)
Zika fever	Zika groznica
Zoonosis	Zoonoza

PHARMACY — **LJEKARNA**

Activated carbon	Aktivni ugljen
Adrenaline	Adrenalin
Aerosol	Aerosol
After meal	Nakon jela
Alcohol	Alcohol
Almond oil	Bademovo ulje
Aminophylline	Aminofilin
Ampicillin	Ampicilin
Ampoule	Ampula
Analgesic (painkiller)	Analgetik
Anesthetic	Anestetik
Antacid	Antacid
Anti-diabetic drug	Antidiabetik
Anti-inflammatory	Protuupalno
Anti-obesity medication	Dijetetsko sredstvo
Antialcoholic drug	Antialkoholik
Antiallergic drug	Antialergik
Antianemic	Antianemik
Antiarrhythmic agent	Antiaritmik
Antibiotic	Antibiotik
Anticoagulant	Antikoagulans
Anticonvulsant	Antiepileptik (antikonvulziv)
Antidepressant	Antidepresiv
Antidiarrhoeal drug	Antidiaroik
Antidote	Antidot
Antiemetic and motion sickness drug	Lijek protiv mučnine i povraćanja
Antihelminthic	Antihelmintik
Antihemorrhagic (hemostatic)	Hemostatik
Antihistamine	Antihistaminik
Antihypertensive drug	Antihipertenziv
Antimalarial drug	Antimalarik
Antimycotic	Antimikotik
Antioxidant	Antioksidans
Antiperspirant	Antiperspirant
Antiprotozoal agent	Antiprotozoik
Antipsychotic	Antipsihotik

Antipyretic	Antipiretik
Antirheumatic drug	Antireumatik
Antiseptic	Antiseptik
Antiserum	Antiserum
Antitoxin	Protuotrov
Antitubercular agent	Antituberkulotik
Antiviral drug	Antivirusni lijek
Aspirin	Aspirin
At noon	U podne
Atropine	Atropin
Bandage	Zavoj
Barbiturate	Barbiturat
Blood pressure meter (sphygmo-manometer)	Tlakomjer
Boric acid	Borova otopina
Bronchodilator	Bronhodilatator
Caffeine	Kofein
Calcium	Kalcij
Capsule	Kapsula
Cardiotonic agent	Kardiotonik
Castor oil	Ricinusovo ulje
Cephalosporin	Cefalosporin
Chamomile	Kamilica
Chemotherapy	Kemoterapija
Chloramphenicol	Kloramfenikol
Chlorine	Klor
Cobalt	Kobalt
Codeine	Kodein
Compress	Oblog
Condom	Prezervativ (kondom)
Contact lenses	Kontaktne leće
Contact lenses cleaning solution	Tekućina za čišćenje kontaktnih leća
Contraceptive	Kontraceptiv
Contraceptive foam	Kontracepcijska pjena
Contraceptive pill (oral contraceptive)	Kontracepcijska pilula
Contraceptive sponge	Kontracepcijska spužva
Copper	Bakar
Corticosteroid	Kortikosteroid
Cotton-wool	Vata
Cytostatic	Citostatik
Dental floss	Zubni konac
Denture cleaning solution	Tekućina za čišćenje umjetnog zubala
Diaphragm (Dutch cap)	Dijafragma
Digestive	Digestiv
Diuretic	Diuretik
Dose	Doza
Drops	Kapi (kapljice)
Drug allergy	Alergija na lijek
Drug side-effects	Nuspojave lijeka
Ear drops	Kapi za uši
Emulsion	Emulzija
Enema (clyster)	Klizma (klistir)
Erythromycin	Eritromicin
Essential oil	Eterično ulje
Expectorant	Sredstvo za iskašljavanje
Eye drops	Kapi za oči
Fentanyl	Fentanil
Foam	Pjena
For external application	Za vanjsku primjenu
Gauze sponge	Gaza
Gel	Gel
Gentamicin	Gentamicin
Glasses	Naočale
Glucose	Glukoza
Gram (gramme)	Gram
Hard contact lens	Tvrda kontaktna leća
Heparin	Heparin
Herbal tea	Biljni čaj
Home pregnancy test	Kućni test za trudnoću
Hormone replacement therapy	Hormonalna nadomjesna terapija
Hot water bottle	Termofor
Hypnotic (soporific)	Hipnotik
Immunoglobulin	Imunoglobulin
Immunosuppressive	Imunosupresiv
In the evening	Na večer
In the morning	U jutro
Incontinence pads (adult diapers)	Pelene za inkontinenciju
Inhalation	Inhalacija
Injection	Injekcija
Insect repellent	Sredstvo protiv insekata
Insulin	Inzulin
Interferon	Interferon
International System of Units	Sustav međunarodnih mjernih jedinica
Iodine	Jod
Iron	Željezo
Jojoba oil	Jojobino ulje
Laxative	Laksativ
Lip balm	Grožđana mast
Liquid powder	Tekući puder
Litre	Litra
Lotion	Losion
Lubricant	Lubrikant
Magnesium	Magnezij
Manganese	Mangan
Medical cannabis	Medicinski kanabis
Medication (remedy, drug)	Lijek
Methadone	Metadon
Microgram	Mikrogram
Milligram (milligramme)	Miligram
Millilitre	Mililitar
Mineral	Mineral
Mineral oil	Mineralno ulje
Molybdenum	Molibden

'Morning -after' pill (postcoital contraception, emergency contraception)	Pilula za "dan poslije" (postkoitalna kontracepcija, hitna kontracepcija)	Soft contact lens	Meka kontaktna leća
		Solution	Otopina
		Spasmolytic	Spazmolitik
		Spermicide	Spermicid
		Spoon	Žlica
Morphine	Morfin	Spray	Sprej
Mosquito repellent	Sredstvo protiv komaraca	Sublingual administration	Pod jezik
Mouthwash liquid	Tekućina za ispiranje usne šupljine	Sugar substitute	Umjetno sladilo
		Sulphonamide	Sulfonamid
Mucolytic	Mukolitik	Sulphur	Sumpor
Muscle relaxant	Miorelaksator	Sunscreen (sunblock)	Sredstvo za zaštitu od sunca
Nasal drops	Kapi za nos		
Needle	Igla	Suppository	Čepić
Nicotine gum	Nikotinska guma za žvakanje	Syringe	Šprica
		Syrup	Sirup
Nicotine patch	Nikotinski flaster	Tablet	Dražeja (tableta)
Non-steroidal antiinflammatory drug	Nesteroidni antireumatik	Tampon	Tampon
		Tetracycline	Tetraciklin
		Thermometer	Toplomjer
Nutrient	Nutritiv	Tincture	Tinktura
Nystatin	Nistatin	Tonic	Tonik
Ointment (fat)	Pomada (mast)	Tooth paste	Pasta za zube
Omega-3 fatty acid	Omega-3 masne kiseline	Tramadol	Tramal
		Urinary antiseptic	Uroantiseptik
On empty stomach (before the meal)	Na tašte	Vaccine	Cjepivo
		Vaginal suppository	Vaginaleta
Opioid	Opijat (opioid)	Vasodilatator	Vazodilatator
Orally	Na usta	Viagra (sildenafil citrate)	Viagra
Overdose	Predoziranje		
Oxycodone	Oksikodon	Vial	Bočica
Paracetamol	Paracetamol	Vitamin	Vitamin
Paraffin	Parafin	Vitamin A (retinol)	Vitamin A (retinol)
Paste	Pasta	Vitamin B1 (thiamin)	Vitamin B1 (tiamin)
Pastille (lozenge)	Tableta za sisanje (pastila)		
		Vitamin B2 (riboflavin)	Vitamin B2 (riboflavin)
Penicillin	Penicilin		
Pharmacist	Ljekarnik	Vitamin B3 (niacin)	Vitamin B3 (niacin)
Phosphorus	Fosfor	Vitamin B4 (adenine)	Vitamin B4 (adenin)
Phytotherapy	Fitoterapija		
Piece	Komad	Vitamin B5 (pantothenic acid)	Vitamin B5 (pantotenska kiselina)
Plaster (adhesive strip)	Flaster		
		Vitamin B6 (pyridoxine)	Vitamin B6 (piridoksin)
Poison	Otrov		
Potassium	Kalij	Vitamin B7 (inositol)	Vitamin B7 (inozitol)
Potion	Ljekoviti napitak		
Powder	Prašak (puder)	Vitamin B8 (biotin)	Vitamin B8 (biotin)
Prescription	Recept	Vitamin B9 (folic acid)	Vitamin B9 (folna kiselina)
Psychostimulant	Psihostimulans		
Purgative	Purgativ	Vitamin B10 (factor-R)	Vitamin B10 (faktor-R)
Rectal	Rektalno		
Rinsing	Ispiranje	Vitamin B11 (factor-S)	Vitamin B11 (faktor-S)
Salicylate	Salicilat		
Saline solution	Fiziološka otopina	Vitamin B12 (cobalamin)	Vitamin B12 (kobalamin)
Sanitary pads (sanitary napkins)	Higijenski ulošci		
		Vitamin C (L-ascorbic acid)	Vitamin C (L-askorbinska kiselina)
Scales	Vaga		
Sedative	Sedativ	Vitamin D2 (ergocalciferol)	Vitamin D2 (ergokalciferol)
Serum	Serum		
Skin cream	Krema	Vitamin D3 (cholecalciferol)	Vitamin D3 (kolekalciferol)
Soap	Sapun		
Sodium	Natrij		

Vitamin D4	Vitamin D4
Vitamin D5 (sitocalciferol)	Vitamin D5 (sitokalciferol)
Vitamin E (tocopherol)	Vitamin E (tokoferol)
Vitamin F (linoleic acid)	Vitamin F (linoleična kiselina)
Vitamin J (choline)	Vitamin J (kolin)
Vitamin K (phylloquinone)	Vitamin K (filokinon)
Vitamin L1 (anthranilic acid)	Vitamin L1 (antranilna kiselina)
Vitamin P (flavonoids)	Vitamin P (flavonoidi)
Water-soluble tablets	Šumeće tablete
Zinc	Cink
Zinc ointment	Cinkova pasta

MEDICAL FACILITIES, PROCEDURES AND CARE — *MEDICINSKE USTANOVE, ZAHVATI I NJEGA*

Administration of drugs	Davanje lijekova
Airway (cannula)	Kanila
Alarm	Uzbuna (alarm)
Ambu bag valve mask	Ambu balon s maskom
Ambulance	Kola hitne pomoći
Ambulance (clinic)	Ambulanta
Amputation	Amputacija
Anesthesia	Anestezija (narkoza)
Arthrodesis	Artrodeza
Artificial respiration	Umjetno disanje
Autopsy	Obdukcija
Balance training	Trening ravnoteže
Bath (wash)	Kupati
Bathroom	Kupaonica
Bed	Krevet
Bed rest	Mirovanje u krevetu
Bite	Zagristi
Blanket	Deka
Blood donation	Darovanje krvi (donacija krvi)
Body positioner	Udlaga za pozicioniranje
Breakfast	Doručak
Breast implant	Umetak za dojku
Breathing exercises	Vježbe disanja
Bypass	Premosnica
Calling of the time of death	Proglašenje vremena smrti
Cardiology	Kardiologija
Catheter	Kateter
Cause of death	Uzrok smrti
Cauterization	Kauterizacija
Chamber -pot	Noćna posuda
Chemotherapy	Kemoterapija
Circumcision	Obrezivanje
Cleansing	Pročišćavanje
Close	Zatvoriti
Contagious	Zarazno
Corpse	Leš
Cover	Pokrivač
CPR mask	Maska za oživljavanje
Crutch	Štaka
Cryoextraction	Krioekstrakcija
Cytology	Citologija
Debris	Otpad (otpadni proizvod)
Defecation	Pražnjenje stolice (defekacija)
Defibrillation	Defibrilacija
Defibrillator	Defibrilator
Dental crown	Zubna krunica
Dental extraction	Vađenje zuba
Dental filling	Zubna plomba
Dentist	Stomatolog (zubar)
Dentures	Umjetno zubalo
Dermatology	Dermatologija
Diagnosis	Dijagnoza
Dialysis	Dijaliza
Die	Umrijeti
Diet	Dijeta
Digestion	Probava
Dining-room	Blagavaonica
Dinner (supper)	Večera
Doctor (physician)	Liječnik
Doctor's office	Liječnička ambulanta
Donor	Davalac (donator)
Door	Vrata
Drain tube	Dren
Drainage	Drenaža
Dressing	Previjanje
Drill	Bušilica
Dynamometer	Dinamometar
Electrode	Elektroda
Electrode conductive gel	Kontaktni gel za elektrode
Electrosurgery	Elektrokirurgija
Electrotherapy	Elektroterapija
Elevator	Dizalo
Emergency medical services	Hitna služba
Endotracheal tube	Endotrahealna kanila
Escape chair	Sjedalica za evakuaciju
Exercise	Vježbanje
Facelift (rhytidectomy)	Lifting lica (ritidektomija)
Feeding tube	Sonda za hranjenje
First aid	Prva pomoć
First aid kit	Kutija prve pomoći
Gastric lavage (stomach pumping)	Ispiranje želuca
General anesthesia	Opća anestezija
General practitioner	Liječnik opće prakse
Germs	Klice

Gerontology	Gerontologija	Ophtalmology ward	Očni odjel
Get changed	Presvući se	Oropharyngeal	Orofaringealna
Goniometer	Goniometar	airway	kanila
Gynecology	Ginekologija	Orthopedics	Ortopedija
Head immobilizer	Imobilizator glave	Otorhinolaryngolo-	Uho-grlo-nos
Health insurance	Zdravstveno	gy	
	osiguranje	Overbed table	Stolić za serviranje
Hearing assist	Slušni aparat		hrane
device		Oxygen mask	Maska za kisik
Heel and elbow	Zaštitnici za pete i	Oxygen storage	Boca s kisikom
protectors	laktove	tank	
Heimlich maneuver	Heimlichov zahvat	Pacemaker	Električni stimulator
(abdominal thrusts)			srca
Hospital	Bolnica	Palpation	Pregled pipanjem
Hospital trolley	Kolica		(palpacija)
Hydrotherapy	Hidroterapija	Pathology	Patologija
Immunology	Imunologija	Patient	Bolesnik
Incontinence pad	Gumirano platno	Patient's room	Bolesnička soba
Infectious disease	Zarazni odjel	Pediatrics	Pedijatrija
unit		Percussion	Pregled kucanjem
Infusion	Infuzija		(perkusija)
Infusion stand	Stalak za infuziju	Percutaneous	Perkutana koronarna
Injection	Injekcija	coronary	angioplastika
Intensive care	Intenzivna njega	intervention	
Intensive care unit	Jedinica intenzivne	(coronary	
	njege	angioplasty)	
Internal medicine	Interna medicina	Pessary	Pesar
Intubation	Intubacija	Physical therapy	Fizikalna terapija
Kegel exercise	Kegelove vježbe	Physiotherapist	Fizioterapeut
Laparoscopic	Laparoskopska	Pillow	Jastuk
surgery	operacija	Plaster cast	Gipsana udlaga
Laryngeal mask	Laringealna maska	(immobilization	
airway		plaster)	
Laryngoscope	Laringoskop	Plastic surgery of	Plastična operacija
Laundry	Vešeraj	the abdomen	trbuha
Light	Svjetlo	("tummy tuck",	(abdominoplastika)
Liposuction	Liposukcija	abdominoplasty)	
Litter bin	Kanta za smeće	Plastic surgery of	Plastična operacija
Liver dialysis	Dijaliza jetre	the breasts	dojke
Lobotomy	Lobotomija	(mammoplasty)	(mastoplastika)
Local anesthesia	Lokalna anestezija	Plastic surgery of	Plastična operacija
Lunch	Ručak	the eyelid	očnog kapka
Manometer cuff	Manšeta tlakomjera	(blepharoplasty)	(blefaroplastika)
Manual de	Ručni defibrilator	Plastic surgery of	Plastična operacija
fibrillator		the nose	nosa (rinoplastika)
Mattress	Madrac	(rhinoplasty)	
Medical center	Medicinski centar	Postural drainage	Drenažni položaj
Morgue (mortuary)	Mrtvačnica	Primary health care	Primarna
Nasal cannula	Nosna kanila		zdravstvena zaštita
Neck immobilizer	Imobilizator vrata	Protect gloves	Zaštitne rukavice
Neurology	Neurologija	Protection cap	Zaštitna kapa
Night table	Noćni ormarić	Protection face	Zaštitna maska za
(bedside table)		mask	lice
Nightgown	Spavačica	Protection gown	Zaštitna navlaka za
Nurse	Medicinska sestra		odjeću
Nursing (care)	Njega	Protection shoe	Zaštitna navlaka za
Occupational	Radni terapeut	cover	obuću
therapist		Psychiatry	Psihijatrija
Oncology	Onkologija	Psychologist	Psiholog
Open	Otvoriti	Pulmonary ward	Plućni odjel
Operating room	Operacijska sala	Pyjamas (pajamas)	Pidžama
Operation (surgery)	Operacija	Quarantine	Karantena

Radiation	Zračenje	Surgical removal of	Kirurško
Radiology	Radiologija	a hemorrhoid (he-	odstranjenje
Reanimation	Oživljavanje	morrhoidectomy)	hemeroida
	(reanimacija)		(hemoroidektomija)
Reception office	Prijemni ured	Surgical removal of	Kirurško
Recipient of an	Primatelj organa	a lobe of some	odstranjenje režnja
organ		organ (lobectomy)	nekog organa
Recover (heal)	Ozdraviti		(lobektomija)
Recovery	Oporavak	Surgical removal of	Kirurško
Rehabilitation	Rehabilitacija	a testicle	odstranjenje testisa
(rehab)		(orchidectomy)	(orhidektomija)
Remission	Stadij mirovanja	Surgical removal of	Kirurško
	bolesti (remisija)	adenoids	odstranjenje trećeg
Renal dialysis	Dijaliza bubrega	(adenoidectomy)	krajnika
Respirator	Aparat za disanje		(adenoidektomija)
	(respirator)	Surgical removal of	Kirurško
Rhinology	Rinologija	one or both adrenal	odstranjenje
Rinse	Isprati	glands	nadbubrežne žlijezde
Scalpel	Skalpel	(adrenalectomy)	(adrenalektomija)
Scissors	Škare	Surgical removal of	Kirurško
Semi -intensive care	Poluintenzivna njega	stones (lithotomy)	odstranjenje
Sheet	Plahta		kamenca (litotomija)
Shunt	Spoj (skretnica)	Surgical removal of	Kirurško
Slippers	Šlape	the aneurysm	odstranjenje
Sonde	Sonda	(aneurysmectomy)	aneurizme
Spit	Pljunuti		(aneurizmektomija)
Sponge	Spužva	Surgical removal of	Kirurško
Sterile (aseptic)	Sterilno	the gallbladder	odstranjenje žučnog
Sterilization	Sterilizacija	(cholecystectomy)	mjehura
Stethoscop	Stetoskop		(kolecistektomija)
Storage	Spremište	Surgical removal of	Kirurško
Stretcher	Nosila	the larynx	odstranjenje grkljana
Suction catheter	Usisni kateter	(laryngectomy)	(laringektomija)
Suction unit	Aspirator	Surgical removal of	Kirurško
(aspirator)		the pancreas	odstranjenje
Surgery	Kirurgija	(pancreatectomy)	gušterače
Surgical opening of	Kirurško otvaranje		(pankreatektomija)
a direct airway on	dišnog puta	Surgical removal of	Kirurško
the neck	(traheotomija)	the prostate gland	odstranjenje prostate
(tracheostomy)		(prostatectomy)	(prostatektomija)
Surgical opnening	Kirurški zahvat	Surgical removal of	Kirurško
of the cranium	otvaranja lubanje	the spleen	odstranjenje slezene
(craniotomy)	(kraniotomija)	(splenectomy)	(splenektomija)
Surgical procedure	Kirurški zahvat	Surgical removal of	Kirurško
of formation of	formiranja stome	the stomach	odstranjenje želuca
stoma (colostomy)	(kolostomija)	(gastrectomy)	(gastrektomija)
Surgical procedure	Kirurški zahvat na	Surgical removal of	Kirurško
on a joint	zglobu (artrotomija)	the thymus	odstranjenje prsne
(arthrotomy)		(thymectomy)	žlijezde
Surgical procedure	Kirurški zahvat na		(timektomija)
on the middle ear	srednjem uhu	Surgical removal of	Kirurško
(stapedectomy)	(stapedektomija)	the thyroid gland	odstranjenje štitne
Surgical procedure	Kirurški zahvat na	(thyroidectomy)	žlijezde
on the spine	kralježnici		(tiroidektomija)
(laminectomy)	(laminektomija)	Surgical removal of	Kirurško
Surgical procedure	Kirurški zahvat na	the uterus	odstranjenje
on the thalamus	talamusu	(hysterectomy)	maternice
(thalamotomy)	(talamotomija)		(histerektomija)
Surgical removal of	Kirurško	Surgical removal of	Kirurško
a breast	odstranjenje dojke	the vermiform	odstranjenje slijepog
(mastectomy)	(mastektomija)	appendix	crijeva
		(appendectomy)	(apendektomija)

Surgical removal of tonsils (tonsillectomy)	Kirurško odstranjenje krajnika (tonzilektomija)
Surgical removal of uterine myomas (myomectomy, fibroidectomy)	Kirurško odstranjenje mioma u maternici (miomektomija)
Surgical sterilization of a man (vasectomy)	Kirurška sterilizacija muškarca (vazektomija)
Surgical sterilization of a woman (tubal ligation)	Kirurška sterilizacija žene (podvezivanje jajovoda)
Table (desk)	Stol
Tea	Čaj
Teeth polishing	Poliranje zuba
Test tube	Epruveta
Therapy	Liječenje (terapija)
Toilet (lavatory)	Nužnik
Traction	Trakcija
Transfusion	Transfuzija
Transplantation	Presađivanje (transplantacija)
Transurethral resection of the prostate	Transuretralna resekcija prostate
Trauma	Trauma
Trendelenburg position	Trendelenburgov položaj
Tweezers	Pinceta
Urination (voiding)	Mokrenje (uriniranje)
Urological catheter	Urinarni kateter
Urology	Urologija
Using a toilet	Obaviti nuždu
Vaccination (inoculation)	Cijepljenje
Vaccination schedule	Kalendar cijepljenja
Vacuum mattress	Vakumirani madrac
Visit	Posjeta
Visitor	Posjetitelj
Vital signs monitor	Monitor za praćenje vitalnih znakova
Waiting -room	Čekaonica
Walker (walking frame)	Hodalica
Ward	Odjel
Wardrobe (cupboard, cabinet)	Ormar
Wash basin	Lavor
Water	Voda
Wheelchair	Invalidska kolica
Window	Prozor
Wound stitching	Šivanje rane

MEDICAL EXAMS	MEDICINSKE PRETRAGE
Abdominal ultrasound	Ultrazvuk abdomena
Agglutination tests	Test aglutinacije
Alkaline phosphatase	Alkalna fosfataza
Alpha -fetoprotein test (AFP test)	Alfafetoproteinski test (AFP)
Amniocentesis	Amniocenteza
Angiography	Angiografija
Anoscopy	Anoskopija
Antibiogram	Antibiogram
Aortography	Aortografija
Arteriography	Arteriografija
Arthroscopy	Artroskopija
Aspartate transaminase (SGOT)	Transaminaze u serumu
Audiometry	Audiometrija
Barium enema	Rendgensko snimanje debelog crijeva i rektuma s kontrastom barija
Barium meal (upper gastrointestinal series)	Rendgensko snimanje želuca i dvanaesnika barijevom kašom
Benzidine stool test	Benzidinski test stolice
Biochemical blood tests	Biokemijske pretrage krvi
Biomarker	Biomarker
Biopsy	Biopsija
Blood culture	Mikrobiološki pregled krvi (hemokultura)
Blood gas test	Analiza plinova u krvi
Blood pressure monitoring	Mjerenje krvnog pritiska
Blood sugar concetration (glucose level)	Šećer u krvi
Blood urea nitrogen test (BUN)	Ostatni dušik u krvi (urea nitrogen test)
Bone densitometry (dual energy X-ray absorpriometry)	Denzitometrija kostiju (apsorpciometrija kostiju)
Bone marrow biopsy	Biopsija koštane srži
Bone scintigraphy	Scintigrafija kostiju
Bone X-ray (bone radiography)	Rendgensko snimanje kostiju
Brain ventricle biopsy	Biopsija moždanih klijetki (ventrikulopunkcija)
Breast examination	Pregled dojke
Breast ultrasound	Ultrazvuk dojke

Bromsulphalein	Brom-sulfalein test
liver function test	funkcije jetre
Bronchography	Bronhografija
Bronchoscopy	Bronhoskopija
CA 125 (cancer	CA 125
antigen 125)	(karcinomski antigen
	125)
CA 19-9	CA 19-9
(carbohydrate	(karbohidratni
antigen)	antigen)
Carcinoembryonic	Karcinoembrionski
antigen (CEA)	antigen (CEA)
Cardiac	Kateterizacija srca
catheterization	(angiokardiografija)
(heart cath,	
angiocardiography)	
Cardiac ultrasound	Ultrazvuk srca
(echocardiography)	(ehokardiografija)
Cardiotocography	Kardiotokografija
Catheter	Kateterska
angiography	angiografija
Central venous	Centralni venozni
pressure (CVP)	pritisak (CVP)
Cephalometry	Cefalometrija
Cerebral	Cerebralna
angiography	angiografija
Cerebrospinal fluid	Pregled likvora
analysis	
Cerebrospinal fluid	Mikrobiološki
culture	pregled likvora
Cervical conization	Konizacija
Chest X-ray	Rendgensko
	snimanje srca i pluća
Cholangiography	Kolangiografija
Colonoscopy	Kolonoskopija
Colposcopy	Kolposkopija
Complete blood	Kompletna krvna
count	slika
Computed	Kompjuterizirana
tomography (CT)	tomografija (CT)
Contrast medium	Kontrast
Coronary	Koronarografija
catheterization	
(coronarography)	
Cystography	Cistografija
Cystoscopy	Cistoskopija
Defecography	Defekografija
Dental X-ray	Rendgensko
	snimanje zuba
Dermatoscopy	Dermatoskopija
(dermoscopy)	(dermoskopija)
Differential	Diferencijalna
diagnosis	dijagnoza
Digital subtraction	Digitalna
angiography	supstrakcijska
	angiografija
Dilated fundus	Pregled očnog
examination	fundusa
DNA analysis	DNK analiza
Doppler	Ultrazvuk srca s
echocardiography	dopplerom
Drug induced	Širenje zjenica
pupillary dilatation	potaknuto lijekovima
Echoencephalogra-	Ehoencefalografija
phy	
Electrocardiogra-	Elektrokardiografija
phy (ECG)	(EKG)
Electroencephalo-	Elektroencefalografi-
graphy (EEG)	ja (EEG)
Electromyography	Elektromiografija
(EMG)	(EMG)
Electroneurography	Elektroneurografija
Electroretinogra-	Elektroretinografija
phy	
Endometrial biopsy	Biopsija endometrija
Endoscopic	Endoskopska
retrograde cholan-	retrogradna kolangi-
giopancreatography	opankreatografija
(ERCP)	(ERCP)
Endoscopy	Endoskopija
Enteroscopy	Enteroskopija
Ergometry test	Test opterećenja
	(ergometrija)
Erythrocyte	Sedimentacija
sedimentation rate	eritrocita
Esophageal	Manometrija
manometry	jednjaka
Esophagogastrodu-	Ezofagogastrodoude-
odenoscopy	noskopija
Fine needle	Punkcijsko-
aspiration biopsy	aspiracijska biopsija
Fluoroscopy	Fluoroskopija
Functional	Funkcionalna
magnetic resonance	magnetska
imaging (functional	rezonancija (FMR)
MRI)	
Gastric juice	Kemijski pregled
chemical	želučanog soka
examination	
Gastroscopy	Gastroskopija
Glasgow coma scale	Glasgowska skala
	kome
Glucose urine test	Šećer u urinu
Gonioscopy	Gonioskopija
Gynecological	Ginekološki pregled
examination	
HbsAg (Hepatitis B	HbsAg (hepatitis B
surface antigen)	površinski antigen)
Hematocrit	Hematokrit
Hepatobiliary	Scintigrafija jetre i
scintigraphy with	žučnih vodova
technetium -99m	radioaktivnim
	izotopima
High intensity	Fokusirani ultrazvuk
focused ultrasound	visokog intenziteta
Hysterescopy	Histeroskopija
Hysterosalpingo-	Rendgensko
graphy	snimanje maternice i
	jajovoda
Indirect Coombs	Indirektni Coombsov
test	test
Intravenous	Intravenozna
biligraphy	biligrafija

Intravenous pyelography	Intravenozna pijelografija (i.v. Urografija)	Pelvigraphy	Rendgensko snimanje zdjelice i porođajnog kanala
Iodine -131 thyroid test	Test štitnjače na provodljivost radioaktivnog joda 131	Pelvimetry	Pelvimetrija
		Perimetry	Perimetrija
		Phenolsulfonphtha-lein test (PSP test)	Fenolsulfoftaleinski test (PSP-test)
Joint X-ray (arthrography)	Rendgensko snimanje zgloba	Phlebography	Venografija (flebografija)
Karyotype	Kariotip	Plethysmography	Pletizmografija
Kidney biopsy	Biopsija bubrega	Pleural biopsy	Biopsija pleure
Laboratory (lab)	Laboratorij	Pneumoencephalo-graphy	Pneumoencefalogra-fija
Laboratory tests	Laboratorijske pretrage	Polysomnography (sleep study)	Polisomnografija (viseparametarski test u pracenju procesa sna)
Laparoscopy	Laparoskopija		
Laryngoscopy	Laringoskopija		
Liver biopsy	Biopsija jetre		
Liver function tests	Funkcionalne pretrage jetre	Positron emission tomography	Pozitronska emisijska tomografija (PET)
Liver ultrasound	Ultrazvuk jetre		
Lumbar myelography	Lumbalna mijelografija	Post-void residual urine volume	Ostatni urin (rezidualni urin)
Lumbar puncture	Lumbalna punkcija	Pregnancy test	Test na trudnoću
Lung scintigraphy	Scintigrafija pluća	Prostate specific antigen	Prostatični specifični antigen (PSA)
Lymph node biopsy	Biopsija limfnog čvora		
Lymphography (ly-mphangiography)	Limfografija	Prothrombin time	Protrombinski indeks
Magnetic resonance imaging (MRI)	Magnetska rezonancija (MR)	Pulmonary angiography	Pulmonalna angiografija
Magnetoencephalo-graphy (MEG)	Magnetoencefalogra-fija (MEG)	Pulse monitoring	Mjerenje pulsa
		Pyelography	Pijelografija (urografija)
Mammography	Mamografija		
Mantoux test (PPD test)	Tuberkulinski kožni test	Radioisotope scanning (nuclear medicine)	Radioizotopna dijagnostika
Mediastinoscopy	Medijastinoskopija		
Microbiological culture	Mikrobiološki pregled (kultura)	Rapid strep test	Brzi test na streptokok (strep-test)
Myelography	Mijelografija		
Ophtalmoscopy	Oftalmoskopija	Rectal examination	Rektalni pregled
Oral cholecystography	Rendgensko snimanje žučnog mjehura s kontrastom (peroralna kolecistografija)	Rectoscopy	Rektoskopija
		Refractometry	Ispitivanje refrakcije
		Renal scintigraphy	Scintigrafija bubrega
		Renal ultrasound	Ultrazvuk bubrega
		Retrograde pyelography	Retrogradna pijelografija
		Rose Waaler test	Rose Waaler test
Oral glucose tolerance test (OGTT)	Oralni test tolerancije na glukozu (OGTT)	Semen analysis	Spermogram
		Serology blood tests	Serološke pretrage na antitijela
Otoscopy	Otoskopija	Serum albumin	Albumin u serumu
Pancreas ultrasound	Ultrazvuk gušterače	Serum bilirubin	Bilirubin u serumu
		Serum protein electrophoresis	Elektroforeza proteina u serumu
Papanicolau test (Pap test)	Papa-test (Papanicolaouova klasifikacija)	Sialography	Sijalografija
		Sigmoidoscopy	Sigmoidoskopija
Partial thromboplastin time (PTT)	Parcijalno tromboplastinsko vrijeme (PTT)	Skin allergy testing (prick test)	Alergološko testiranje kože (prick test)
Patch test	Kožni alergološki test flasterom	Skin biopsy	Biopsija kože
		Skull X-ray (craniography)	Rendgensko snimanje lubanje
Patellar reflex	Patelarni refleks		

Speech audiometry	Govorna audiometrija	X-ray (radiography)	Rendgen
Spinal angiography	Spinalna angiografija	**PREGNANCY**	
Spine X-ray (spine radiography)	Rendgensko snimanje kralježnice	**AND OBSTETRICS**	**TRUDNOĆA I PORODNIŠTVO**
Spirometry (vital capacity test)	Spirometrija (mjerenje vitalnog kapaciteta)	Abortifacients Abortion (pregnancy	Abortivni lijekovi Prekid trudnoće (abortus)
Spleen scintigraphy with technetium	Scintigrafija slezene radioaktivnim	termination) Absence of	Izostanak mjesečnice
-99m	izotopima	menstrual period	(amenoreja)
Sputum culture	Mikrobiološki pregled ispljuvka	(amenorrhea) Amniocentesis	Amniocenteza
Stereotactic biopsy	Stereotaktična biopsija	Amnioscopy Amniotic fluid	Amnioskopija Plodna voda
Suboccipital myelography	Subokcipitalna mijelografija	Amniotic sac	(amnijska tekućina) Vodenjak
Suboccipital puncture	Subokcipitalna punkcija	Artificial insemination	Umjetna oplodnja
Thoracoscopy	Torakoskopija	Biological parent	Biološki roditelj
Throat swab culture	Mikrobiološki pregled brisa grla	Biophysical profile of the fetus	Biofizikalni profil fetusa
Thyroid biopsy	Biopsija štitnjače	Birth canal	Porodni kanal
Thyroid blood tests	Test na hormone štitnjače u krvi	Blastocyst Bleeding	Blastocista Krvarenje
Thyroid scintigraphy	Scintigrafija štitnjače	(haemorrhage) Body length of a	(hemoragija) Dužina
Thyroid ultrasound	Ultrazvuk štitnjače	newborn	novorođenčeta
Tomography	Tomografija	Braxton Hicks	Lažni trudovi
Tonometry	Tonometrija oka	contractons	
Transthoracic percutaneous fine	Perkutana transtorakalna	Breast Breast pump	Dojka Pumpica za izdajanje
needle aspiration	punkcija pluća	Breathing	Disanje
Tumor marker	Tumorski marker	Breech	Zadak
Tympanocentesis	Timpanocenteza	Breech position	Stav zatkom
Tympanometry	Timpanometrija	Cardiotocography	Kardiotokografija
Ultrasound (medical	Ultrazvuk	Cervical dilation	Otvaranje ušća maternice
ultrasonography)			
Ultrasound of the gallbladder and bile	Ultrazvuk žuči i žučnih vodova	Cesarean section (C-section)	Carski rez
ducts		Chadwick's sign	Hiperemična
Urea breath test	Urea izdisajni test		sluznica rodnice
Urea clearance test	Urea klirens		(Chadwickov znak)
Ureteroscopy	Ureteroskopija	Childbirth	Porod
Urethrography	Uretrografija	Choriocarcinoma	Koriokarcinom
Urine chemical	Kemijska analiza	Chorion	Korion
analysis	urina	Chorion-	Korion-gonadotropin
Urine culture	Mikrobiološki pregled mokraće	gonadotrophin Chorionic villi	Korionske resice
	(urinokultura)	Chorionic villus	Uzorak korionskih
Urine protein test	Bjelančevine u urinu	sampling	resica
Urine specific	Specifična težina	Conception	Začeće (oplodnja)
gravity	urina	Contracted pelvis	Sužena zdjelica
Urobilinogen in	Urobilinogen u urinu	Cordocentesis	Kordocenteza
urine		Curettage	Kiretaža
Vaginal swab	Mikrobiološki	Cut	Presjeći
culture	pregled brisa rodnice	Delivery room	Rađaona
Ventriculography	Ventrikulografija	Diaper	Pelena
Weber test	Weberov test	Dizygotic twins (biovular twins)	Dvojajčani blizanci

Duration of contraction	Trajanje truda	Inflammation of the fetal membranes (chorioamnionitis)	Upala plodovih ovoja (korioamnionitis)
Duration of pregnancy	Trajanje trudnoće	Inflammation of the urinary bladder (cystitis)	Upala mokraćnog mjehura (cistitis)
Eclampsia	Eklampsija		
Ectopic pregnancy (extrauterine pregnancy)	Izvanmaternična trudnoća (ektopična trudnoća)	Inner membrane of the uterus (endometrium)	Sluznica maternice (endometrij)
Edema	Edem	Intensity of contractions	Snaga trudova
Egg donation	Donacija jajašca		
Ejaculation	Ejakulat	Intracytoplasmatic sperm injection	Intracitoplazmatska spermalna injekcija
Embryo	Embrij (zametak)		
Endometrial hyperplasia	Hiperplazija maternice	Labor contraction frequency	Frekvencija trudova
EPH gestosis (preeclampsia)	EPH-gestoze (preeklampsija)	Labor contractions	Trudovi
Episiotomy	Kirurško proširenje porođajnog kanala (epiziotomija)	Lactation	Dojenje (laktacija)
		Lactiferous duct	Mliječni vod
		Leg varicose veins	Proširene vene na nogama
Excessive secretion of saliva (hypersalivation)	Pojačano lučenje sline (hipersalivacija)	Lithopedion (stone baby)	Litopedion (okamenjeno dijete)
Expulsion of placenta	Istiskivanje posteljice i ovoja	Lochia	Lohija (iscjedak u babinjama)
Expulsion of the baby	Istiskivanje ploda	Macrosomia (big baby syndrome)	Fetalna hipertrofija
Fallopian tube (oviduct)	Jajovod	Maternity blues (baby blues)	Labilno psihičko raspoloženje (baby blues)
Father	Otac		
Fetal anomalies (fetal abnormalities)	Anomalije fetusa	Maternity hospital	Rodilište
		Meconium	Mekonij
Fetal hypotrophy	Fetalna hipotrofija	Meconium aspiration syndrome	Mekonijalni aspiracijski sindrom
Fetal pH-metry	Fetalna pH-metrija		
Fetal weight (birth mass)	Težina ploda (porođajna težina)		
		Meconium ileus	Mekonijalni ileus
Fetoscopy	Fetoskopija	Meconium peritonitis	Mekonijalni peritonitis
Fetus	Fetus		
Forceps	Forceps (kliješta)	Medically assisted procreation	Medicinski potpomognuta oplodnja
Full term birth	Ročni porod		
Gestational diabetes	Gestacijski dijabetes		
Graafian follicle	Graafov folikul	Medication that suppresses premature labor (tocolytic)	Lijek za sprečavanje trudova (tokolitik)
Gynecology	Ginekologija		
Habitual abortion (recurrent miscarriage)	Habitualni pobačaj		
		Menopause	Menopauza (klimakterij)
Head	Glavica		
Hemolytic disease of the newborn	Hemolitička bolest novorođenčeta	Menstrual cycle	Menstruacijski ciklus
High blood pressure (hypertension)	Visoki krvni tlak (hipertenzija)	Menstruation	Menstruacija
		Microcephaly	Mikrocefalija (sitnoglavost)
Hymen	Djevičnjak (himen)		
Hypertrophy of uterus	Hipertrofija maternice	Midwife	Babica
		Mifepristone	Mifepriston
Implantation	Implantacija (usađivanje)	Monozygotic twins (identical twins)	Jednojajčani blizanci
In vitro fertilisation	Oplodnja in vitro	Morula	Morula
Incubator	Inkubator	Mother	Majka
Infection	Infekcija	Multigravida	Višerotkinja
Infertility	Neplodnost (sterilitet)	Multiple pregnancy	Blizanačka trudnoća
		Nausea	Mučnina
		Navel (belly button)	Pupak
		Neck	Vrat

Neonatology	Neonatologija	Spermatozoon	Spermij
Newborn (infant)	Novorođenče	(sperm cell)	
Nipple	Bradavica	Spontaneous	Spontani pobačaj
Nuchal scan (nuchal	Nuhalna	abortion	
translucency)	translucencija	(miscarriage)	
Obstetrician	Porodničar	Stage of birth	Porodno doba
	(opstetičar)	Stillborn	Mrtvorođenče
Obstetrics	Porodništvo	Suckling	Sisanje
Oogenesis	Ovogeneza	Surgical removal of	Kirurško
	(oogeneza)	the uterus	odstranjenje
Ovarian hyperemia	Hiperemija jajnika	(hysterectomy)	maternice
Ovary	Jajnik		(histerektomija)
Ovulation	Ovulacija	Surrogate mother	Surogat majka
Ovum	Jajašce	(womb mother)	(zamjenska majka)
Parent	Roditelj	TORCH infections	TORCH infekcije
Pathological birth	Patološki porod	Transverse fetal	Kosi položaj ploda
Pelvimetry	Pelvimetrija	position	
Placenta	Posteljica (placenta)	Twins	Blizanci
Placenta accreta	Prirasla posteljica	Ultrasound	Ultrazvuk
	(placenta acrreta)	(medical	
Placenta previa	Placenta previja	ultrasonography)	
Placental abruption	Abrupcija posteljice	Umbilical cord	Pupkovina (pupčana
Placental estrogen	Estrogen placente		vrpca)
Placental	Progesteron placente	Umbilical cord	Ispala pupkovina
progesterone		prolapse	(prolaps pupkovine)
Plagiocephaly	Plagiocefalija	Urinary	Urinarna
Postmature birth	Poslijeročni porod	incontinence	inkotinencija
Postnatal	Babinje (puerperij)	Urinary retention	Zastoj urina
(postpartum		(ischuria)	(urinarna retencija)
period,		Uterine anomalies	Anomalije maternice
puerperium)		Vacuum extractor	Vakuumski
Postnatal	Postporođajna	(ventouse)	ekstraktor
depression	depresija	Vagina	Rodnica
(postpartum		Vomiting	Povraćanje
depression)		Water birth	Porod u vodi
Postpartum	Puerperalna psihoza	Womb (uterus)	Maternica (uterus)
psychosis			
Pregnancy	Trudnoća		
Pregnancy risk	Teratogeni faktori		
factors	rizika		
Premature birth	Prijevremeni porod		
Premature rupture	Prijevremeno		
of membranes	prsnuće vodenjaka		
Preterm newborn	Nedonošće		
Primigravida	Prvorotkinja		
Progesterone	Progesteron		
Prolactin	Prolaktin		
Prolonged birth	Produljeni porod		
Puerperal fever	Puerperalna groznica		
	(babinja groznica)		
Puerperal mastitis	Puerperalni mastitis		
Puerperal sepsis	Puerperalna sepsa		
Push	Tiskati		
Pyelonephritis	Pijelonefritis		
Quadruplets	Četvorci		
Rupture of	Prsnuće vodenjaka		
membranes			
Semen (sperm)	Sjemena tekućina		
	(sperma)		
Sperm bank	Banka sperme		
Sperm viability	Životna sposobnost		
	spermija		

ABOUT THE AUTHOR

Edita Ciglenečki is medical translator with Academic degrees in Biomedical Sciences and Public Health Sciences. Besides Croatian, being her mother tongue, she is a holder of international diplomas in English, French and Italian language. For many years she worked as a medical professional inside the travel industry. This dictionary is the product of her own working experience built on her passion for travelling, medicine and language skills.